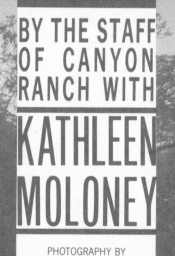

BY THE STAFF
OF CANYON
RANCH WITH

KATHLEEN
MOLONEY

PHOTOGRAPHY BY
JEANNE STRONGIN

SIMON AND SCHUSTER

NEW YORK LONDON TORONTO SYDNEY TOKYO

THE
CANYON RANCH HEALTH
AND
FITNESS PROGRAM

SIMON AND SCHUSTER
Simon & Schuster Building
Rockefeller Center
1230 Avenue of the Americas
New York, New York 10020

Copyright © 1989 by Sabino Health & Fitness Resort, Inc.
All rights reserved
including the right of reproduction
in whole or in part in any form.

canyon ranch ®

CANYON RANCH is a registered trademark of
Sabino Health & Fitness Resort, Inc.
SIMON AND SCHUSTER and colophon are registered trademarks
of Simon & Schuster Inc.

Designed by Bonni Leon
Photographs on pp. 107–110 by Leslie Lindig
Manufactured in the United States of America

10 9 8 7 6 5 4 3 2 1
Library of Congress Cataloging in Publication Data

The Canyon Ranch health and fitness program / by the staff of the
    Canyon Ranch, Kathleen Moloney.
        p.   cm.
    Includes index.
        1. Health.   2. Physical fitness.   I. Moloney, Kathleen.
    II. Canyon Ranch.
    RA776.C23   1989   88-33358
        613—dc 19   CIP

ISBN 0-671-66116-7

This book is dedicated to the memory of Norman Zuckerman, who was the inspiration for Canyon Ranch, and to all people—past, present, and future—who don't want to end their lives saying, "I wish I had done it differently."

CONTENTS

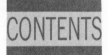

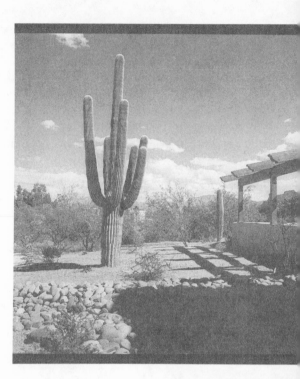

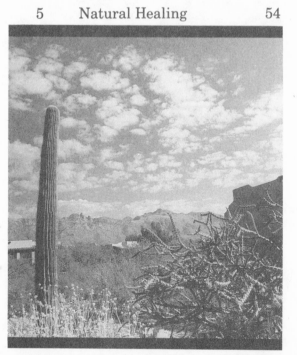

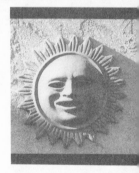

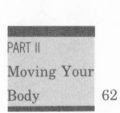

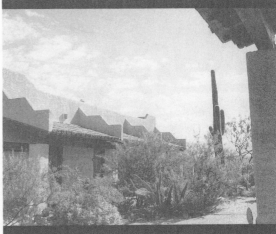

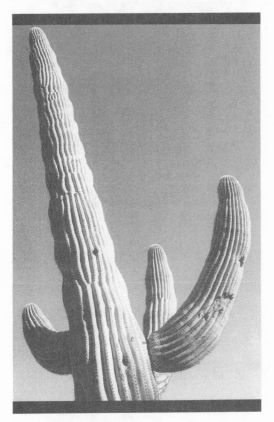

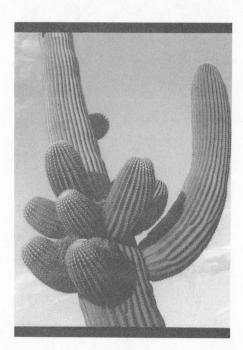

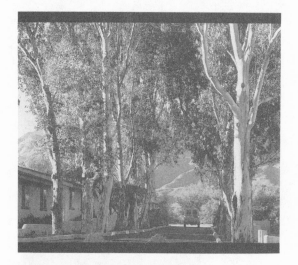

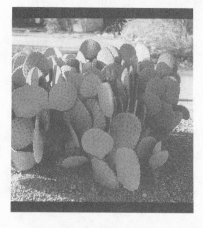

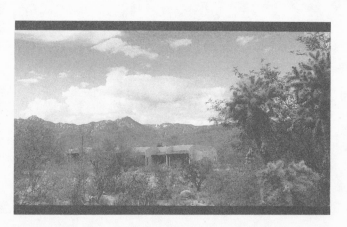

ACKNOWLEDGMENTS

Most Canyon Ranch projects are collaborative efforts, and this book is no exception. The material in it is the product of the thoughts, opinions, expertise, passions, and favorite stories of many people. Some of their names appear in the book, but we'd like to take this space to thank all of the people who helped Mel and Enid Zuckerman and the writer make this book a reality.

Our thanks go to Jerry Cohen, president and chief financial officer; Bill Day, chief operating officer; Dan Baker, executive director of health services; Karma Kientzler, executive director of fitness services; Jack Stern, the Ranch's first medical director, and Phil Eichling, the current medical director; Ron Limoges, head of the Canyon Ranch Foundation; Jeanne Jones, food consultant and developer of the Canyon Ranch menu; and Leah Kovitz, skin care director. They all gave most generously of their time.

Our thanks go as well to Andrew Weil and Deborah Morris, who discussed holistic medicine and natural healing; V. V. Hughes, Mary Deits, and Kevan Schlamowitz, who shared their expertise about stress management; Julie Kembel, who offered facts and insights about food habit management and the Stop Smoking Program; dietitians Linda Connell and Mary Perry, who gave of their expertise in nutrition; and Sheila Wagner and Karen Wedding, who provided additional information about tests and other medical matters.

Much of the exercise physiology information was provided by Gary Holzsager, Eric Chesky, and Denise Gater. Others who talked about specific fitness areas are Phyllis Hochman, Meredith Wittwer, Annette Fair, Lynne Pray Raugh, Mary Margaret Walmer, Coco Fell, Bev Elliott, Kathy Foster, Joe Turk, and Frank Lister.

Lynn Kerry, Rose Marie Martin, Lina Williams, and Roni Kendall provided information about massage, Kim Weers talked about how the Canyon Ranch program works at home, and Alison Limoges discussed the creative arts. Brian Shultz, Michael LaBoeuf, Donna Kreutz, Carolyn Niethammer, Kevin Alexander, Connie LaPaglia, Marian Tripp, Kathy Draper, and Cindy Hintze helped to coordinate it all.

But before any of that happened, Ron Taub, a Chicago businessman and a consultant to Canyon Ranch, and Charles Hayward, now president of Simon & Schuster, came up with the idea for this book over a vigorous game of tennis in the Tucson sun; agent Dominick Abel worked out the details; and editor Carole Lalli helped with the fine-tuning. We thank them all.

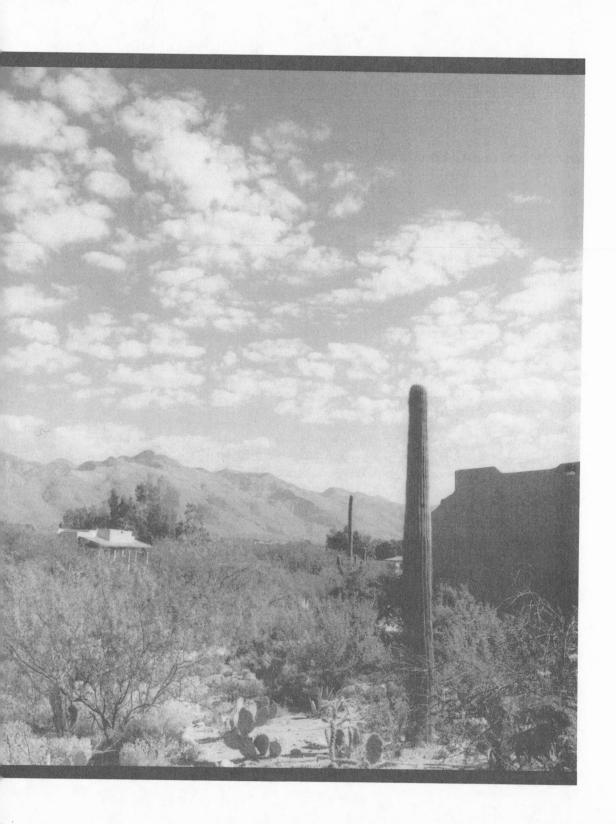

FOREWORD

"YOU CANNOT TEACH A PERSON ANYTHING. YOU CAN ONLY HELP HIM FIND IT FOR HIMSELF."
—GALILEO

In August of 1977 my father died of cancer. He'd been a two-pack-a-day smoker all his life, and my mother and I had spent nearly thirty years trying to get him to stop. Sometimes we succeeded, and he would quit for a day or two or five; but he just couldn't kick the habit. Then one day, when he was 76 years old, his doctor told him he had a spot on his lung. Then and there, in the doctor's office, thirty seconds after he learned he had lung cancer, my father crumpled a pack of cigarettes in his hand and said, "I quit." And he did. Even so, my mother and I buried him eleven months later.

My father and I were in business together, so I saw him almost every day of that eleven months. At least once a day during that time he would wander into my office, sit on the corner of my desk, and say, "If only I had stopped sooner . . ." or "I wish I'd listened to you . . ." or "Do you think I can beat this thing?" My father had had a good life, but at 76, he wasn't ready to die. He wanted more. And he was tortured by the fact that he had commissioned his own death.

I turned 50 the year my father died, and until then I don't think I had ever faced my own mortality. Watching him die, listening to him talk about what he should have done, was the worst experience I'd ever had, and it taught me the most important lesson I'll ever learn: health may not be everything, but if you don't have your health, you don't have anything. I promised myself then and there that I was not going to let what happened to my father happen to me. I was not going to spend the last year of my life saying, "If only . . ."

To put it mildly, I had my work cut out for me. At 50 years old I weighed 210 pounds (about 40 more than I should have), and I was truly the man

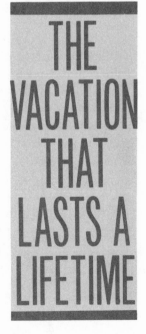

THE VACATION THAT LASTS A LIFETIME

who had everything: asthma, high blood pressure, hiatal hernias, ulcers, and diverticulitis. I worked 16 hours a day and didn't have the stamina to manage even a set of doubles tennis. Determined to change my life, I did what millions of others have done before me—I made a New Year's resolution. On January 1 I vowed that I would lose the 20 pounds my doctor had been nagging me about. By the first of March I had gained four pounds and the depressing realization that I just couldn't do it alone.

A magazine ad for a California spa caught my eye. "Lose a pound a day with Sheila," it said, and it went on to describe the wonders of The Oaks at Ojai. I figured I'd spend ten days there, lose ten pounds with Sheila, and learn a little something about eating. At the end of ten days I had lost 13 pounds and was running a mile and a half in 12 minutes—I who used to huff and puff after walking a few blocks. What's more, I felt as good as I had ever felt in my life, better even than I had in my twenties. At 50 I was doing things I was told I couldn't do in my teens.

Transformed by the high of my new-found feeling of well-being, I called my wife Enid back home in Tucson and told her I had decided to stay a while. In the four weeks I spent at The Oaks I lost 29 pounds and continued to feel healthier and better than I had ever felt in my life. I was deliriously happy. I wanted to feel that good after I went home to Tucson and every day for the rest of my life. Eighteen months later, on December 20, 1979, Enid and I opened the doors of what we had decided to call The Canyon Ranch Spa.

A great deal has been written about the many kinds of spas that have sprung up around the country in the last ten years. There seems to be a place to suit every taste—fasting, rebirthing, allergy detection, weight loss, homeopathic healing, skiing, swimming, even skeet shooting. There are hotels with modest spa facilities, luxurious pamper preserves, spiritual retreats, European-style therapeutic spas, and health crisis centers. As far as I'm concerned, there are no bad spas; there are only bad matches. If you get what you need from your spa experience, it's the right one for you.

Hardly a day goes by that we don't examine the aims and goals of Canyon Ranch, asking ourselves what we are and what we hope to be. We know we're not a fat farm, although it's true we've helped hundreds of people shed more than a few pounds. We know we're not a place where lazy people come to lie around all day and be pampered, although we believe that giving yourself some kind of break from the day's stresses— with a massage, a facial, meditation, deep breathing, an herbal wrap, or just 10 minutes of peace and quiet—is as important for your health as keeping your abdominal muscles firm. In 1982 *Time* magazine published a story about the Ranch that said we "balance the triangle of life," meaning body, mind, and spirit. We were happy with that description.

In the nine years the Ranch has been open we've learned a great deal, not only about every aspect of fitness but also about what motivates people, what makes them want to make significant changes in their lives. Everyone who comes here has a different story, of course. For the 200 guests we have at any one time there are probably 75 reasons for showing up on our doorstep. Some are grieving over the loss of a loved one; some are fighting addictions or recovering from illness; some are overworked and overweight; some are burned out; some are great in business, but they can't seem to get control over the rest of their lives; some have time for everything but eating right and exercise; some want to quit smoking or lower their cholesterol and blood pressure; some are just plain beat.

No matter what the story is, after a week at Canyon Ranch just about everyone loses weight and fat, lowers cholesterol and blood pressure, becomes stronger, more flexible, and more aerobically fit, and decreases the risk factors for heart attack. All that is good news, of course, and it makes for some very satisfied customers. But the even better news is that everyone who comes to Canyon Ranch gets a chance to be reminded of what I discovered years ago back at The Oaks—just how good a healthy life can make you feel. Far from the pressures of the outside world, the guests here find out how good it feels to live well—to exercise, to nourish their bodies sensibly, to relax, and to be taken care of. As surprised as they are by this realization, they are even more stunned at how short a time it takes to feel so much better.

At the Ranch we definitely try to teach. Our physicians, nurses, dietitians, physiologists, fitness instructors, and behavioral and wellness counselors instruct our guests in the ABCs of total fitness, beginning with the rudiments of good nutrition, sensible exercise, and stress management. But changing your life takes more than learning why saturated fats are bad for you and how to do a perfect push-up. It takes a heartfelt belief that what you do makes a difference. We want people to exercise three or four times a week for a half-hour not because it makes the heart muscle stronger and increases oxygen use—though, of course, it does—but because their bodies feel better when they do. We want people to discover that a well-balanced regimen of nutritious meals, regular exercise, and deep relaxation makes them feel better than they've felt in years.

If I eat a pint of ice cream (and believe me, I have been known to), I know it won't kill me. After all, my cholesterol level is okay, and I'm not fat anymore. However, I also know that it will make my nose run and I'll feel generally lousy the next day. It's my choice to make, my responsibility to myself and for myself. Of all the things people learn here at the Ranch the most important is to accept responsibility for their health and well-being, to understand that they can be in control if they choose to be.

A few years ago I was passing the registration desk late at night and I ran into Glen, one of our frequent guests. Glen is a great guy and a very successful businessman, but he was about 75 pounds overweight and gaining fast. His doctor had told him he was heading straight for a heart attack if he didn't change his ways. When I ran into him, he had just arrived and was really feeling down.

"Mel, I'm telling you, I can't beat this thing," Glen said. "I can't stop eating. I swear I hear voices in the middle of the night, telling me to wake up and go down to the kitchen to eat a half a gallon of ice cream. Not a bowl of ice cream, mind you, but a half-gallon." I looked him straight in the eye and told him that if he didn't stop listening to voices and start listening to reason, he—and the voices—would soon be dead.

My response may seem callous, especially since I know very well how strong the call of ice cream can be, but what I said to Glen was true, and I thought it's what he needed to hear. I wanted to shake him up, to make him understand that "voices" are not in charge of his life; he is. That's the message we try to convey to everyone we see here.

Where your health is concerned, you can be either an active participant or a re-active participant. It's your choice. Most of us are oblivious to the consequences of our actions, believing that if we ignore a problem, it will go away. We deny our vulnerability, even our mortality. Until the doctor actually sits us down and gives us bad news, as he did to my father, we aren't motivated to make changes. We're willing to gamble and hope that we won't become a statistic, that we'll be one of the lucky ones who doesn't get cancer or have a stroke or come down with a debilitating disease by the time we reach sixty-five. When we acknowledge the consequences of our actions, it becomes easier to make sensible decisions and take responsibility. We open up more often to the other possibilities, ones that have nothing to do with losing weight and exercising.

Like you, all the people we see here every day have excelled at something in their lives. In fact, the only failure many people have ever had is not being able to quit smoking or lose 15 pounds. We try to make them understand that their success in other areas didn't happen by accident; it took commitment and discipline, the same sort of commitment and discipline you need to stop gorging on chocolate, keep up your swimming program, and learn to stop grinding your teeth. You don't leave your business or your marriage or your social life to chance. Why leave the management of your health and well-being to chance?

Over the years we've seen our share of "miracles"—weight loss, remarkable recoveries from arthritis, diabetes, ulcers, heart disease, and severe emotional trauma—and while each miracle is unique, there is one thing that they all have in common: it was the guests themselves who made it happen. They did it by taking a look at themselves and deciding, then and there, that they wished to make a change. We gave them the tools and a comfortable environment in which to learn how to use them. Then we sent them off to practice what they learned in the Real World.

Yes, I know that Canyon Ranch is not the Real World. We're a cocoon, where every choice you make is a good one and there are no candy machines or deadlines. Here no one smokes or drinks alcohol, there is no caffeine, and everything is designed to support a healthful lifestyle. Here the utmost thing in everyone's mind is maintaining health and well-being; out there many people don't give it a thought. Life at Canyon Ranch is not everyday reality, though we wish it were.

I also know that not everyone can be our guest at the Ranch (I wish that weren't so, either). We feel we have a strong message to spread, and we'd like a big audience to hear it. And that's the reason behind the book you now hold in your hand, so that even without making your way to Tucson you can take advantage of what we've learned. Here are the tools you need to live the kind of life you want for yourself. All of our experts have contributed material, which represents the cutting edge of the fitness and preventive health movement. It covers the latest in nutrition, exercise, stress management, and relaxation techniques, and it includes information related to our special programs, such as Stop Smoking, Food Habit Management, and MindFitness. You have a lot of choices to make about how to live your life. I hope and believe that this book will enhance your health consciousness and help you make informed choices and support you in your commitment. In short, I think the book is the next best thing to being here.

One of the maxims I've come to embrace is, "Wellness is not a destination. It's a journey." I'm on that journey, and I will be all my life. In the last ten years I've changed my life dramatically—I'm healthier today than I was ten years ago—but I still can't have ice cream in the house, and as everyone who knows me will be glad to tell you, I have a lot to learn about managing stress. But step by step, I'm making my way. I hope you'll join me.

—Mel Zuckerman

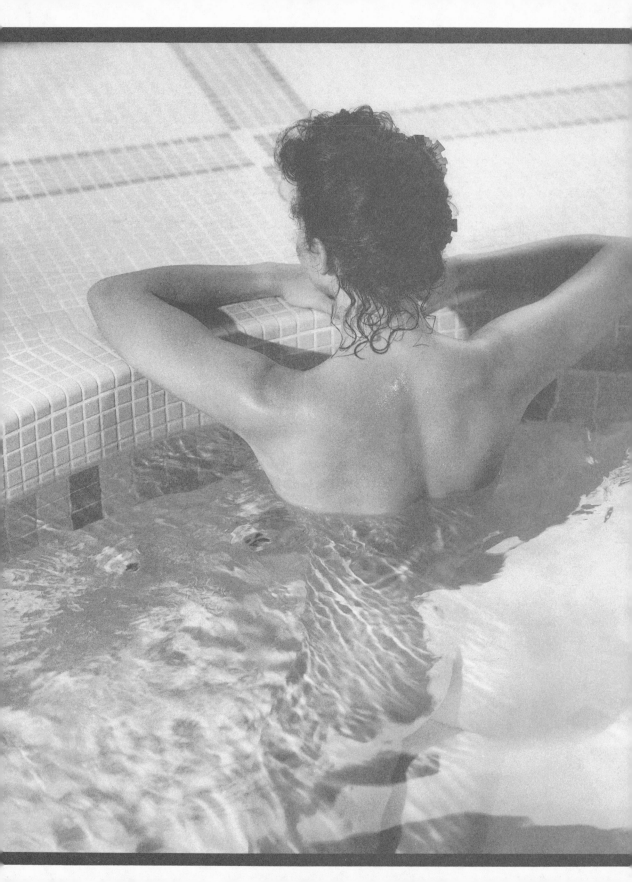

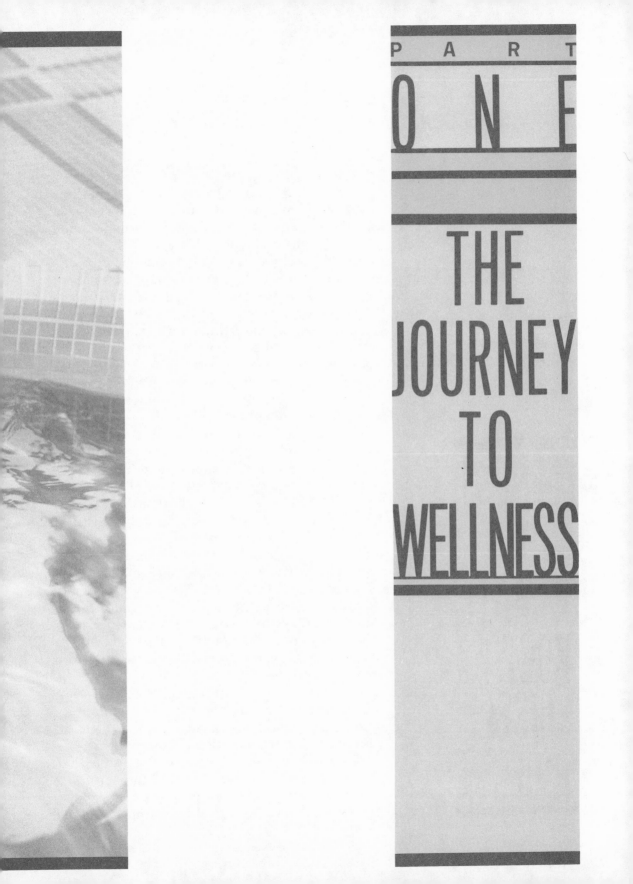

THE JOURNEY TO WELLNESS

WELLNESS: THE ULTIMATE DO-IT-YOURSELF PROJECT

Imagine this scene. You're in your doctor's office. You've just had a thorough checkup, and you're a little nervous about the results of the examination. Your mind is racing. You're sure you've put on a little weight. What if your cholesterol count is too high? The doctor is probably going to bug you about your smoking again. After a few minutes the doctor arrives, sits at his desk across from you, gives you a long, hard look, and says, "Joe/Joan, the way it stands now, you're going to die in five years. However, if you quit smoking, lose ten pounds, and lower your cholesterol by 35 points, you can live for 15 years. If you do that and walk for 40 minutes four times a week, I'll make it 20."

Granted, this scenario is a little far-fetched, but it's only a slight exaggeration of what could, and perhaps *should*, be taking place in doctors' offices all over the country every day. If you don't believe it, pick a study—any study. The medical profession estimates that somewhere between 50 and 90 percent of all illness, disease, and premature death in this country is preventable. The Paffenbarger study (released in 1986 but conducted from the mid-1960s to the late 1970s) shows that more than half of the deaths caused by cardiac failure in this country could have been prevented. Emory University recently identified the 14 primary causes of illness and premature (meaning before age 65) death for which preventive action can be taken; included on the list are infectious diseases, infant mortality, drug abuse, cardiovascular disease, and cancer, which account for about 80 percent of the deaths in the United States.

The Paffenbarger study also suggested that moderate, regular exercise is vital to health and indeed probably prolongs life. Regular exercise appears to reduce the risk of dying from any of the major diseases. Hypertensives who exercise regularly reduce their death rate by half. Furthermore, the more a person exercises, the longer he seems likely to live.

There are other, equally impressive studies and statistics, but they all add up to the same thing: even without any miracles of modern science, even without cures for cancer or the common cold, we can turn ourselves into a much healthier society. We can keep ourselves from getting sick, even make ourselves well; the way we do that is through prevention.

AN OUNCE OF PREVENTION

Our biggest, most widespread health problem today is bad habits. As difficult as it is to accept, to a great extent how we live determines when we will die and what will eventually kill us. Smoking, drinking to excess, consuming high-fat, low-fiber diets, and getting too much sun can lead to hypertension, stroke, heart disease, diabetes, emphysema, and cancer of the skin, breast, colon, or lungs. And all of these life-threatening illnesses are due to choice, not chance. Treating these diseases doesn't seem to be working very well; it's obvious that the best way not to die from one of those diseases is not to get it in the first place.

No one is sure exactly how or how often prevention works. Some people believe that health is all "mind over matter," that if you keep yourself fit and have the right attitude, you can ward off any disease or illness. Others say that getting sick is just a matter of bad luck. The medical journals are filled with debates about whether cancer is preventable through diet or whether exercise stimulates the immune system or whether warding off stress adds years to your life. The complete answers are still to come, but so far it seems clear that prevention doesn't hurt, and it probably helps.

People in our Western culture are not, by nature, inclined to embrace the concept of prevention. We're much more likely to wait until there is trouble, at which time it may well be too late. "If it ain't broke, don't fix it!" we say, and much of the time we're right. When it comes to our health and well-being, however, we're wrong. Prevention suggests ways of decreasing the chances that it will "break," of preventing problems before they start. The goal is to live as properly and healthfully as you can and hope that you don't develop a disease. And in doing so you must begin to emphasize "wellness" instead of illness.

THE ELEMENTS OF WELLNESS

Although the concept of wellness has been around for years, and though it has been widely accepted as a legitimate approach to health, many people still think of it as a trendy buzzword, surrounded by permanent quotation marks. It makes people squirm a little, perhaps out of fear that voodoo is about to be practiced. Some people are put off because wellness, unlike illness, is not easily defined.

Wellness is not the absence of illness, any more than pleasure is the absence of pain. Wellness is much more; it is the sense of well-being that comes from being emotionally alive, physically active, and mentally alert and of having command and control over your own life. There are five basic elements of wellness, each of which is crucial to the whole. Although some of the elements are more traditionally understood—especially the first two—no one element is more important than any other.

♦ Nutritional awareness. This doesn't mean knowing how to gain or lose weight or how many calories are in a piece of cheese or a medium-sized apple. It's being aware of what your body needs to fuel and nourish it so that it functions most comfortably and efficiently.

♦ Physiological awareness. Again, this does not mean committing to memory exactly how many calories are burned when you do aerobic exercise. It involves a working knowledge of the basic components of physical fitness and an appreciation of how much and what kind of exercise your body needs to work best.

♦ Mental development. An understanding of the outside stimuli that are likely to cause you anxiety or stress or interfere with productive thinking and a working knowledge of any of a number of techniques, such as deep breathing and meditation, that you may call upon to stimulate and relax you.

♦ Environmental attunement. An ability to stand back from the immediate worries of the world—job, family, social life, whatever—and become more aware of and appreciate the appeal of the natural world.

♦ Realization of the dream. Some say that the ultimate barometer of our well-being has to do with our ability to rebound from trauma and our ability to realize our dreams, to achieve that which makes our hearts sing and makes us feel the joy of being alive. Many of us, caught up in the more mundane goals of our lives, can barely remember what that dream is.

Embracing wellness means much more than being able to run a 10K race or fit into a pair of size 8 shorts. It's more than keeping your cool in a traffic jam. It means realizing that you and you alone are responsible for your health, fitness, and systemic balance and learning to be sensitive to your body and aware when something goes wrong. Wellness comes with the knowledge that you are doing everything in your power to diminish your risk of disease, slow down your body's degenerative processes, and make choices that will enhance your life.

Although the word wellness may continue to scare off a few people in some quarters (sometimes they feel better when we call it "optimal health"), there is no question that the concept is catching on. One of the first questions we ask all of our guests at Canyon Ranch is, "Why have you come here?" Nine years ago, when we opened, eight out of ten people answered, "To lose weight." These days weight loss is far from the most popular reason. Now the hands shoot up most often when we ask how many people want a better sense of balance and control in their lives. What they want, whether they use the word or not, is wellness.

GETTING MOTIVATED

Prevention all seems so simple, doesn't it? All we have to do is identify the things that are bad for us and stop doing them, and we won't get sick. Of course, it's anything but simple. Many of us don't wear seat belts and don't examine our breasts and don't quit smoking and don't lose weight. Why do the Surgeon General and the highway patrol and the American Heart Association seem to care more about our health than we do?

One reason is ignorance; we don't know about the dangers until it's too late. After all, it takes years of smoking and a terrible diet to develop heart disease or cancer. Another is that we're experts at kidding ourselves. We think we'll live forever, that it's always the other guy who gets sick. And then, of course, we don't get much support in our efforts to live a healthy life; we live in a society that in many ways encourages us to smoke, drink, and eat junk food. Perhaps the most perplexing reason for our refusal to make changes is that we have dangerously short memories. How many people who have had heart attacks continue to smoke cigarettes and pile on the pounds? When the pain starts, they promise never to smoke again and never to get within forking distance of a piece of cake, but the minute they leave the hospital, they renège on their promises and revert to their bad behavior. Once the pain is gone, the memory fades.

Fear can be a strong motivator. Every day we talk to people who've had a scare: the 52-year-old accountant who was told that if he didn't lose 30 pounds and lower his cholesterol by 100 points, he would be dead in a year or the 34-year-old teacher whose doctor said that her arthritis would eventually cripple her completely. But the formless fear of dying is not always enough, particularly if the only way we can make the fear go away is to give up something we like. It's one thing to understand intellectually that you have to make changes in your life. It's another to have the awareness "click" and to make the commitment to do it. (For more about habits and how to break them see Chapter 4.)

GETTING STARTED

Quit smoking, cut out fried foods and ice cream, get regular exercise, and don't have more than two drinks a day. Those are just a few of the "tips" we're used to seeing and hearing when we hear about leading healthier lives. There is nothing wrong with those tips or any of a hundred others—in fact, you'll find many in this book—but before you get to that stage, you have to have a *plan*. Wellness is a process by which you make changes, large and small, that will prevent disease and promote good health. You need an approach to living that evolves one day at a time and one choice at a time. Here's our nine-step program.

1 Take charge. Realize that you can and must take responsibility for your own health. Most illnesses can be prevented or significantly improved if you live right. No one but you can do it.

2 Take stock. Make some decisions about the quality of your life. Longevity is a wonderful thing, but much more important than how long you live is how you spend the years you have. Your goal should be to live as healthy and active a life as you can manage. Ask yourself what you want your life to be like—mentally, physically, emotionally, and spiritually—in five years. If you are honest, you will probably come to realize that you need to make some changes.

3 Know yourself. See your doctor for a thorough medical check-up and make it your business to understand what the results mean (see Chapter 2). Know what you should weigh and what your blood pressure and cholesterol count are and should be and get to know the conditions under which you're likely to experience stress. Identify and understand your risk factors for disease and learn about your particular problem areas.

4 Educate yourself. After you know which areas need improvement, learn exactly what you can do to reverse the damage that has been done or prevent additional problems. If you need to lower your cholesterol or blood pressure, learn precisely how to do it. Find out whatever you need to know about nutrition and exercise and stress

management. You can't fix the problem if you don't know what you're doing. Don't be like the diabetic who, when told he had to avoid sugar, switched to powderless jelly doughnuts.

5 Don't kid yourself. Set realistic goals. Most people can't look like fashion models or run a marathon in 2:30 no matter what they do; after all, you can't fight genes and body types. Challenging or pushing yourself a little can be good, but setting yourself up for failure can be a disaster. Do the best you can with what you've got.

6 Take it slow. Make all changes, big or small, slowly and gradually. If you try to go too fast, you'll just get frustrated. Don't get hung up on numbers on the scale or mileage on your pedometer. If you stick to a sensible program, you'll get results.

7 Make friends with moderation. Don't be too tough on yourself. There's no point in depriving yourself of everything you like (except cigarettes, which *must* go) or setting up a diet, exercise, or stress management regimen that's virtually impossible to stick to. Moderation may not be the most exciting thing in the world, but when it comes to making behavioral changes, it's the only thing that works.

8 Don't think of your new habits as temporary. Try not to regard it as "going on a diet" or "joining a health club for six months." Think of your new, healthy habits as part of a way of life that you're going to continue forever.

9 Expect setbacks. Brace yourself for imperfection and understand that a bad choice is not a disaster; it's just a bad choice. Only when it leads to other bad choices does it do any real harm to the long-term process of change.

HOW TO USE THIS BOOK

It's time now to think about your plan for improving the quality of your life. In the chapters that follow we'll take you through the process step by step. In Part I you'll learn how to talk to your doctor in plain English and how to interpret the results of a check-up; how to assess your risk factors for disease and the actions you can take to lessen the risks; how to break habits; and how to expand your thinking about alternative medicine. Part II covers exercise, including the benefits of the three basic kinds and advice about the best way to set up your own program. In Part III we talk about food—what's good, what's bad, and how you can manage your habits so that you eat more of the former and less of the latter. Part IV examines stress and how to manage it and provides information about breathing exercises, yoga, biofeedback, hypnotherapy, and other relaxation techniques. In Part V we talk about the importance of pampering yourself and describe some of the most effective ways we know of doing it. Part VI tells you how to keep to a fitness program when you're traveling; how to stop smoking; and how to cook the way we do at the Ranch.

At Canyon Ranch we take our new guests through orientation, asking them about their health, their wellness goals, and their problems and frustrations. We ask them to bring to us a willingness to discover an awakening of mind, body, and spirit. Then we tell them what their choices are and point them in the right direction, helping them to ease out of bad old habits and embrace new, healthful ones. We encourage them to stop looking outside themselves for the solutions to their problems and to look inward instead.

This book is your orientation. As you go through each section, think of wellness as the ultimate do-it-yourself project. Assemble the tools you need for the goals you set and learn the techniques that will make the job easier. Of course, there are no guarantees that you'll live longer or stay well for the rest of your life, but you can be sure that a commitment to wellness will improve the years that you have. Surely that is payoff enough.

I f there is one thing we love in this country, it's measuring things. From report cards to fitness reports to "Test Your Travel IQ" quizzes in the Sunday supplements to mail order handwriting analysis, we love being evaluated and finding out how we stack up against others. In our passion to quantify we keep track of our temperature, our automobile mileage, and anything else we can think of.

And the world is more than happy to oblige us. Advanced technology has made it possible for us to get tested for practically everything; it's getting so that practically every shopping mall you visit offers you a chance to have your blood pressure or your bone density checked. At the Ranch we do believe that there is such a thing as too much testing (and that shopping malls are not the best place to have tests done), but all in all, measurements can be very useful in determining progress or alerting us to trouble. At Canyon Ranch we encourage all our guests to take time out from their exercise classes and saunas to spend a half-hour or so in the nurse's office. After all, you can't very well decide to solve a problem unless you know you have one.

Having tests is one thing. Interpreting the test results is something else again. What does it all mean?

Weight

The National Institutes of Health says that if you exceed your desirable weight by 20 percent, you are seriously endangering your health. What the NIH doesn't tell us, however, is precisely what your desirable weight is. In fact, no one has yet come up with a sure-fire way to determine that

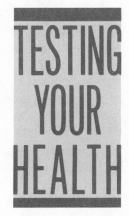

TESTING
YOUR
HEALTH

magic number. Standard height-weight tables give us a starting place, but they're usually out of date. (The most frequently used table, put out by the Metropolitan Life Insurance Company, is about ten years behind the times.) Another problem is that tables don't take into account several factors that may affect weight—family history, race, and age, for example. Many experts say that modest weight gain as you age is perfectly healthy.

Still, we remain hopelessly attached to that number on the scale, and it would be futile to suggest that we throw it out completely. What you should do is understand that your desirable weight is a range, not a precise measurement, and that those numbers must be kept in perspective. Take them for what they're worth in your overall wellness plan.

BODY FAT COMPOSITION

About a year ago a 23-year-old woman, a computer programmer who is fairly athletic, walked into one of our exercise physiologists' offices for a consultation. At 5 feet 6 inches tall she weighed 226 pounds—clearly more than she should. She had made the decision to lose weight, and she told the physiologist, Gary Holzsager, that she was determined to get down to 140. Gary knew from experience (and from the evidence of his own eyes) that the young woman's goals were unrealistic. Yes, the weight tables said that 140 is achievable for someone of her height, but he still didn't think she could—or should—bring her weight down that far. To him 170 sounded about right.

When the determined young woman started to give him an argument, Gary took her through the ABCs of body composition. He started with the assumption that the lowest body fat she could probably manage was 15 percent, on the low side for the average woman her age. If she did reach her goal of 140, he went on to explain, 119 pounds of that (85 percent of 140) would be lean body mass—bones, organs, muscles, and so on. That's the minimum. Then he took her back to her current 226 pounds. If you subtract the 119 pounds of lean body mass from that number, you find that she is carrying 107 pounds of fat, or 47 percent body fat (107 divided by 226). It seemed unlikely to Gary that she was carrying that much fat. To strengthen his case he did a body composition test and discovered that in fact the overweight woman was 35 percent body fat. That means that the day she walked into the office she was carrying 147 pounds of lean body mass (65 percent of 226). It also means that she couldn't possibly weigh as little as 140 without losing lean body mass. She ended up resetting her sights on 170 pounds with 25 percent body fat.

Not too long after that Gary talked to a 37-year-old man whose story had a different kind of ending. When he checked into the Ranch, the man thought that, at 199 pounds, he had about 12 pounds to shed to be in pretty good shape. After his consultation and body composition test, he realized that 12 pounds wouldn't quite do it. It turns out that 31 percent of his current 199 pounds was fat, which is anywhere from 13 to 19 percentage points too high. Instead of getting depressed when he found out that he was in worse shape than he thought, he revamped his plan, eventually losing 36 pounds and reducing his body fat to 13 percent.

WHAT IT MEANS

Body composition is not just an opportunity for physiologists to show off their mathematical prowess. It can be a useful tool and a valuable teaching aid. It can keep people from setting unrealistic goals or kidding themselves. Scale weight is not a true reflection of your health. It's not how much you weigh that matters; it's how fat you are.

Naturally there's a correlation between being overweight and being overfat; if you're obese, you almost certainly have a higher percentage of body fat than you should. (The heavier you are, the less reliable the measurements are.) And there are some contradictions: many football players and body builders are surprisingly low in body fat; chronic dieters can be underweight and overfat. Two people of the same height can have very different weights because of the body fat composition. Even if you weigh the same as you did 20 years ago, you are very probably "fatter" than you were then. A sedentary person will lose about a half a pound of lean weight per year and gain a half pound of fat weight per year from the age of 25 on, which is why your clothes don't fit quite the same even though your weight hasn't changed since high school.

There's no question that measuring body fat has a certain trendiness about it (it sometimes seems as if "What's your body fat?" is destined to take the place of "What's your sign?"), and no doubt the number is occasionally overused. However, when figured into an overall health plan it can be indispensable, particularly when people have a mistaken idea of what their ideal weight is or are thinking of embarking on an unorthodox diet. For instance, one of our guests had been put on a high-protein, low-carbohydrate diet, and we couldn't talk him out of it, especially since he was losing a lot of weight quite quickly. We were worried that he was losing muscle instead of fat, so we suggested that he keep a close watch on his lean mass-fat ratio. After monitoring his body fat for a few months he was persuaded that he was losing the "wrong" kind of pounds.

HOW THE TEST IS DONE

The body-fat composition test is done in one of several ways. The "gold standard" is the hydrostatic weighing method, which is based on Archimedes's principle of water displacement. You sit in a chair in a vat of water, exhale all the air from your lungs, and stay relaxed and motionless submerged in the water for five to ten seconds as the density of your body is weighed. Many people don't care for this method, since getting wet can be inconvenient and the whole procedure of sitting in the chair underwater can cause a bit of anxiety.

The other popular method, the one we use at the Ranch, is the skinfold test, in which a pinch of skin is pulled away from your body and the skinfold between the fingers (skin and subcutaneous fat) is measured with calipers. Most facilities take measurements two or three times—always down the right side of the body—in anywhere from three to six locations and then compute the average. At Canyon Ranch we do both the three-skinfold and the five-skinfold test and average the two results.

Here's where the six measurements are taken:

♦ Subscapular—on the back below the shoulder blade.

♦ Tricep—midway down the back of the arm.

♦ Chest—half way from the armpit to the nipple (for men only).

♦ Suprailiac—top front of the hip.

♦ Abdominal—just off to the side of the belly button.

♦ Thigh—on the front of the thigh approximately a third to halfway down the femur.

Body-fat composition tests are not an exact science. The hydrostatic test comes within about 2 percent accuracy, and the skinfold has a variance of 1 to 3 percentage points. That means that you could be tested one day at 22 percent, the next day at 19, and the day after that at 25.

RECOMMENDED LEVELS

There's also nothing very scientific, or at least very consistent, about the recommended levels of body fat. You'll see recommendations of anything from 6 to 24 percent for men and 9 to 30 percent for women, depending on whose you look at. At the Ranch we recommend 15 to 20 for men and 20 to 26 percent for women. The "high-risk level," which means you're more likely to have a stroke or develop diabetes, heart disease, and cancer, is above 25 percent for men and above 30 percent for women. That is also where mild obesity begins.

Just as you should not let yourself be a slave to the scale, don't be blindly governed by the results of a body-fat composition test. Even if you can achieve a 10 percent body fat, you may feel a lot better at 15. Remember, national averages and statistics are not in charge of your life. You are. And be sure not to have the body fat composition test done too often. You probably won't see any substantial changes in less than a month; wait at least three and preferably six months between tests.

BODY MASS INDEX

Just when you thought it was safe to put your calculator away, there's yet another way to figure out how fat you really are, by computing your body mass index. Simply stated, your body mass index is the figure you get by dividing your weight in kilograms by the square of your height in meters. Let's take it one step at a time:

1. Weigh yourself on the scale. To convert your weight from pounds to kilograms, divide your weight in pounds by 2.2.

2. Measure your height in inches. To convert your height to meters divide that number by 39.4.

3. Square the number of meters and divide the number of kilograms by that number. That gives you your body mass.

For men, the desirable body mass is 22 to 24; above 28.5 is considered overweight, and anything above 33 is considered seriously overweight. The desirable body mass index for women is 21 to 23. Overweight begins at 27.5; anything above 31.5 is thought to be seriously overweight.

BLOOD PRESSURE

An inflatable cuff is wrapped around your arm. Air is then pumped into the cuff until your arterial circulation is cut off; when a stethoscope is placed over the artery cuff, the person taking your blood pressure can't hear anything. Then, as the air is slowly let out of the cuff, blood begins to flow again, mercury begins to rise in a tube, and sound can be heard through the stethoscope. The doctor or nurse records the number that the mercury has reached when the first sound is heard. That number is your *systolic* pressure, and it measures the amount of pressure in your arteries just after the heart has pumped.

As more and more air is let out, the mercury drops, and eventually there is silence once again; the number the mercury reaches when nothing can be heard is your *diastolic* pressure—the pressure in the arteries between heartbeats, when the heart is relaxed.

For example, a systolic reading of 120 means that the mercury is raised to a height of 120 millimeters, and a diastolic reading of 70 means that the mercury reaches a height of 70 millimeters. Your blood pressure reading is thus recorded as 120/70.

Both systolic and diastolic numbers are medically important, but experts tend to pay a bit more attention to the diastolic, because it's less subject to fluctuation. Current research says that the "ideal" blood pressure is 120/80, but a reading as low as 90/70 is usually acceptable. Anything over 140/90 may indicate that there is a problem. Don't let one bad reading scare you, though. If there is cause for concern, you'll need to have it tested again, perhaps several times under different conditions.

Most people have their blood pressure measured dozens, perhaps hundreds, of times in their lives. The blood pressure test is probably the most frequently administered of all diagnostic tests and one of the three tests that determines if your heart is healthy. (The others are the electrocardiogram and the cardiac stress test, described below.) For the doctor who treats you a blood pressure reading offers an excellent way of keeping track of your overall health.

ELECTROCARDIOGRAM

As much as Valentine's Day makes us believe otherwise, the heart is a muscle, and that muscle is composed of hundreds of thousands of individual cells, which produce electricity. Put as simply as possible, an electrocardiogram—often called an EKG—measures the electrical currents produced by the heart. It also determines your heart rate and whether the rhythm is regular or irregular. What an EKG does not tell you is anything about the capacity of your heart.

Unless you have other symptoms of heart disease—particularly an irregular heartbeat—you will probably not find it necessary to undergo an electrocardiogram.

CARDIAC STRESS TEST

The most reliable and most common cardiac stress test is the treadmill test, which monitors the activity of your heart—your EKG, your blood pressure, and your heart rate—as you walk rapidly on a motorized treadmill. The test is relatively simple, but it may make you feel like something out of the "Six Million Dollar Man"; ten electrodes are connected on one end to a monitor and on the other to your body by means of adhesive pads.

The cardiac stress test is administered to evaluate your cardiac status for any of several reasons. The most common are:

♦ if you're about to embark on a fitness regimen after a long period of inaction;

♦ if you've had symptoms of heart disease, such as chest pain, dizziness, palpitations, or unrelieved indigestion;

♦ if your doctor has reason to believe you have a high risk of developing heart disease;

♦ if you're involved in a cardiac rehabilitation program.

BLOOD TESTS

No one particularly enjoys having blood drawn, but there is no way around the fact that many vital pieces of information can be gotten only by blood tests conducted in a laboratory. A thorough blood examination, which we do at the Ranch as part of our Prevention Series, includes 29 different work-ups, including an analysis of cholesterol, glucose, and kidney, liver, and thyroid functions. When the results come back from the lab, we take our guests through the results test by test, pointing out problem areas, if there are any, and recommending solutions.

As you can imagine, many people think that what we tell them is more (maybe a *lot* more) than they need to know. Even if they don't say so, we can tell they're bored when we see their eyes glaze over somewhere between Albumin and Hematocrit. Still, we think it's important to have at least some understanding of what the numbers on that printout mean.

The Canyon Ranch laboratory profile includes basic chemistries, blood count, thyroid studies, and a urinalysis. The purpose of these tests is to screen guests for disease, but we also use them to educate. In discussing the test results we talk about preventable diseases, such as diabetes, hypertension, and cholesterol problems.

Here's a sample readout of the blood test results we show our guests, complete with the range of acceptable levels for each of the tests (see page 32).

Here is a very brief explanation of what each test measures.

♦ Cholesterol. This is a measurement of the fat in your blood. The jury is still out on the ideal cholesterol reading, but the consensus is that anything under 200 is acceptable and 150 to 180 is optimal. Total cholesterol is then broken down into three parts: HDL (high-density lipoprotein) cholesterol; LDL (low-density lipoprotein) cholesterol; and VLDL (very low-density lipoprotein) cholesterol.

♦ HDL. The higher the HDL, the better off you are. A range of 30 to 80 is acceptable, and anything over 50 is considered very good.

♦ LDL. With LDL it's the other way around: the lower the number is, the healthier you are likely to be. The acceptable range is 80 to 185; anything under 100 is considered good.

TEST	UNITS	NORMAL RANGE*
GLUCOSE	MG/DL	70–115
SODIUM	MMOL/L	136–145
POTASSIUM	MMOL/L	3.5–5.0
CHLORIDE	MMOL/L	99–110
BUN	MG/DL	10–26
CREATININE	MG/DL	0.7–1.5
BUN/CREAT RATIO	—	7.1–28.6
URIC ACID	MG/DL	2.2–7.7
CALCIUM	MG/DL	8.5–10.5
IN. PHOSPHATE	MG/DL	2.5–4.5
ALK PHOSPHATASE	U/L	30–115
G. G. T. P.	U/L	0–60
BILI, TOTAL	MG/DL	0.0–1.2
SGOT (AST)	U/L	0–41
SGPT (ALT)	U/L	0–45
LDH	U/L	100–230
CHOLESTEROL	MG/DL	140–229
TRIGLYCERIDES	MG/DL	30–160
PROTEIN, TOTAL	G/DL	6.0–8.5
ALBUMIN	G/DL	3.0–5.5
GLOBULIN	G/DL	2.1–3.6
A/G RATIO	—	1.1–2.0
IRON	MCG/DL	40–160
HDL CHOLESTEROL	MG/DL	30–80
LDL CHOLESTEROL	MG/DL	80–185
VLDL CHOLESTEROL	MG/DL	8–72
TOTAL CHOL/HDL RATIO	—	4.5–5.5
% HDL CHOLESTEROL	—	16–46
WHITE BLOOD CELLS	THOUS/CU. MM.	4.5–10.6
RED BLOOD CELLS	MIL/CU. MM.	4.2–5.6
HEMOGLOBIN	G/DL	12.0–16.0
HEMATOCRIT	%	37–47
MCV	FL	82–103
MCH	PG	27–34
MCHC	G/DL	32.5–35.7
RDW	—	11.5–14.5
PLATELET COUNT	THOUS/CU. MM.	130–440
GRANULOCYTES	%	43–85
LYMPHOCYTES	%	10–47
MONONUCLEAR CELLS	%	0–10
T3 UPTAKE	%	25–35
T4 (THYROXINE)	MCG/DL	4.8–12.3
T7 INDEX	—	1.2–4.3

* The ranges noted apply to a 40-year-old female.

♦ VLDL. This measures Very Low Density Lipoprotein, another constituent of the fats in the blood.

♦ Total cholesterol/HDL ratio. The last number to be considered is your total cholesterol count divided by your HDL. (For instance, if your total cholesterol is 160 and your HDL is 40, your cholesterol/HDL ratio is 4:1. The average man has a reading of 4:1 to 5:1, and the average woman is 4:1 to 4.5:1. Anything under 3.5:1 for men and 3.2:1 for women puts you in the lowest risk category for heart disease.

♦ Glucose. This measures sugar in your blood; it is a test for diabetes.

♦ Sodium, potassium, and chloride. These are the salts in the blood, vital to the muscles and heart.

♦ Bun, Creatinine, Bun/Creat Ratio. These are kidney function tests.

♦ Uric Acid. If a uric acid reading is above the recommended level, you're at a high risk for gout.

♦ Calcium and Phosphorus. This measures the calcium and phosphorus in the blood, as opposed to the bones. (It is not a test for osteoporosis, despite what it sounds like.)

♦ Alk Phosphatase, GGTP, Bili, Sgot, Sgpt, and LDH6. These are liver tests, which determine if your liver has been injured, especially as a result of alcohol or drug consumption.

♦ Triglycerides. Another kind of blood fat.

♦ Protein. A protein deficiency in the blood is quite rare; it appears only in people with extremely inadequate diets or in geriatric patients.

♦ White Blood Counts. White blood cells are the ones that fight infection. This test evaluates the immune system and tests for leukemia.

♦ Iron, Red Blood Counts, Hematocrit, MCV, and MCH. Tests for anemia.

THE HEALTH RISK APPRAISAL

At Canyon Ranch the "Health Risk Appraisal" form is the closest thing we have to a crystal ball. Once a guest has answered the questions on the form and after the results of the cholesterol and blood pressure test have been factored in, we can look into the future. First we analyze your current health status and your habits; then we do a statistical analysis of your risk of dying from the 12 most common causes of death compared to others of your age: breast cancer, heart attack, lung cancer, stroke, cancer of the ovaries, cervix, or intestines, cirrhosis, diabetes, suicide, motor vehicle accidents, and non-motor vehicle accidents. Finally, we put it all together and give you your "health age," explaining, for example, that

HEALTH RISK APPRAISAL

NAME _____

DATE _____

Are you being treated for high blood pressure? _____

Are you being treated for heart disease? _____

Please list medications you are taking for either of the above conditions:

_____

Circle answers unless indicated   Birthday (month) _____ **(day)** _____ **(year)** _____

1. SEX   [1] Male   [2] Female

2. RACE/ORIGIN   [1] White (non-Hispanic   [2] Black (non-Hispanic   [3] Hispanic
                         origin)   origin)
                     [4] Asian or Pacific   [5] American Indian or   [6] Not Sure
                         Islander   Alaskan Native

3. AGE (At Last Birthday)   Years Old □□

4. HEIGHT (Without Shoes)   Example: 5 foot, 7½ inches 5' 08" = [5]' [0][8]"   □' □□"

5. WEIGHT (Without Shoes)   Pounds □□□

6. TOBACCO   [1] Smoker   [2] Ex-Smoker   [3] Never Smoked
  SMOKERS: Enter average number smoked per day during   Cigarettes Per Day   □□
             the last five years.   Pipes/Cigars Per Day (Smoke Inhaled)   □□
                                               Pipes/Cigars Per Day (Smoke Not Inhaled)   □□

  EX-SMOKERS: Enter average number smoked per day during
                the last five years before quitting.   □□
  (Ex-smokers only) Enter Number of Years Stopped Smoking (Note: Enter 1 for less than one year)   □□

7. ALCOHOL   [1] Drinker   [2] Ex-Drinker   [3] Non-Drinker (or drinks less
                                                         than one drink per week)
  DRINKER Enter the average number of drinks per week.   Bottles of beer per week   □□
  EX-DRINKER Enter the average number of drinks per   Glasses of wine per week   □□
           week consumed before you quit drinking.   Mixed drinks or shots of liquor per week □□

8. DRUGS/MEDICATION How often do you use tranquilizers?
                   [1] Almost every day   [2] Sometimes   [3] Rarely or Never

9. MILES Per Year as a driver of a motor vehicle and/or passenger of
         an automobile (10,000 = average)   Thousands of miles □□[0][0][0]

10. SEAT BELT USE (percent of time used)
              Example: about half the time = [5] [0]   □□□ %

11. PHYSICAL ACTIVITY LEVEL

[1] Level 1 = little or no physical activity
[2] Level 2 = occasional physical activity
[3] Level 3 = regular physical activity at least
3 times per week

NOTE: Physical activity includes work and leisure activities that require sustained physical exertion such as walking briskly, running, lifting, and carrying.

12. Did either of your parents have or die of a heart attack before the age of 60?
[1] Yes, One of them   [2] Yes, Both of them   [3] No   [4] Not sure

13. Did your mother, father, sister, or brother have diabetes?   [1] Yes   [2] No   [3] Not Sure

14. Do YOU have diabetes?
[1] Yes, not controlled   [2] Yes, controlled   [3] No   [4] Not sure

15. **Rectal problems** (other than piles or hemorrhoids)
Do you have or have you had any of the following:

Rectal Growth?	[1]	Yes	[2]	No	[3] Not sure
Rectal Bleeding?	[1]	Yes	[2]	No	[3] Not sure

Does a physician examine your rectum annually?   [1] Yes   [2] No   [3] Not sure
(either a finger exam or a proctoscopic exam)

16. Has your physician ever said you have *chronic* Bronchitis or Emphysema?
[1] Yes   [2] No   [3] Not sure

17. **Blood Pressure** (if known - otherwise leave blank)

Systolic (High Number) ☐☐☐
Diastolic (Low Number) ☐☐☐

18. Fasting Cholesterol Level   MG/DL ☐☐☐

19. Considering your age, how would you describe your overall physical health?
[1] Excellent   [2] Good   [3] Fair   [4] Not Sure

20. In general how satisfied are you with your life?
[1] Mostly Satisfied   [2] About Average   [3] Mostly Disappointed   [4] Not Sure

21. In general how strong are your social ties with your family and friends?
[1] Very Strong   [2] About Average   [3] Weaker than Average   [4] Not Sure

22. How many hours of sleep do you usually get at night?
[1] 6 hours or less   [2] 7 hours   [3] 8 hours   [4] 9 hours or more

23. Have you suffered a serious personal loss or misfortune in the Past Year? (For example, a job loss, disability, divorce, separation, jail term, or the death of a close person)
[1] Yes, one serious loss   [2] Yes. Two or more serious losses   [3] No

24. How often in the Past Year did you witness or become involved in a violent or potentially violent argument?

[1] 4 or more times [2] 2 or 3 times   [3] Once or never   [4] Not Sure

25. How many of the following things do you usually do?
- Hitch-hike or pick up hitch-hikers
- Carry a gun or knife for protection
- Keep a gun at home for protection
- Criticize or argue with strangers
- Live or work at night in a high-crime area
- Seek entertainment at night in high-crime areas or bars

[1] 3 or more   [2] 1 or 2   [3] None   [4] Not Sure

26. Have you had a hysterectomy? (Women only)

[1] Yes   [2] No   [3] Not Sure

27. How often do you have Pap Smear? (Women only)

[1] At least once per year [2] At least once every 3 years [3] More than 3 years apart

[4] Have never had one [5] Not sure   [6] Not applicable

28. Was your last Pap Smear Normal? (Women only)

[1] Yes   [2] No   [3] Not sure   [4] Not applicable

29. Did your mother, sister, or daughter have breast cancer? (Women only)

[1] Yes   [2] No   [3] Not Sure

30. How often do you examine your breasts for lumps? (Women only)

[1] Monthly   [2] Once every few months   [3] Rarely or never

31. Have you ever completed a computerized Health Risk Appraisal Questionnaire like this one?

[1] Yes   [2] No   [3] Not Sure

32. **Current Marital Status** [1] Single (Never married) [2] Married [3] Separated
[4] Widowed [5] Divorced [6] Other

33. **Schooling completed** (One choice only)
[1] Did not graduate from high school [2] High School
[3] Some College [4] College or Professional Degree

34. **Employment Status** [1] Employed [2] Unemployed
[3] Homemaker, Volunteer, or Student [4] Retired, Other

35. **Type of occupation** (SKIP IF NOT APPLICABLE)
[1] Professional, Technical, Manager, Official, or Proprietor [2] Clerical or Sales
[3] Craftsman, Foreman, or Operative [4] Service or laborer

36. **County of Current Residence** (SKIP IF NOT KNOWN)

while you may have the birth certificate of a 46-year-old, you have the body of a 56-year-old.

All this may seem a bit cold-blooded, and in many ways it is. It is also one of the most effective ways we know to shake people up. It's one thing to feel guilty about carrying around some extra poundage and never getting any exercise. It's something else again to discover that you have a 75 percent chance of dying of a heart attack before your sixtieth birthday.

One man who visits the Ranch regularly says that the Health Risk Appraisal affected him as nothing, not even a father who died of heart disease at an early age, ever had before. "I had high blood pressure and was taking medication for it, but otherwise I thought I was really healthy," he said. "I was overweight, but I was really quite strong, and I play hours of killer racquetball every week. But then I got the results of my tests. It turns out my cholesterol level was way over 300, and my blood pressure was still out of sight. I'm only 50, but my tests said I may as well be 60.

"That interview changed my life. In six months I lost 40 pounds and brought my cholesterol down to 120. I no longer have to take blood pressure medication. I'm now four years 'younger' than my real age. I've just about reached my achievable health age."

A vital part of the health risk appraisal is the time we spend talking about your achievable health age, how many years you can add to your life by making changes in your life. That's when you learn that all is not lost, that if you change your ways—bring down your blood pressure, get a regular Pap smear, quit smoking, examine your breasts every month, and use your seat belt, for example—you can add years to your life.

When all is said and done, these and other tests are just tools, indicators of what you must do to become healthier. Of course, all the tests in the world won't improve your health or lengthen your life. Only you can do that.

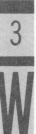

3

e all know the stereotype of the heart attack victim: a cigar-smoking male executive with a large belly and a short fuse. Like most stereotypes, this one has an element of truth to it, but it doesn't come close to telling the whole story. The fact is that heart disease, the number-one killer in the United States today, can affect anyone.

It does seem to strike some people more often than others, as the Framingham study, which has been tracking the health habits and the health of about 5000 people in that Massachusetts town for 35 years, discovered. They determined that heart disease sufferers had one or more conditions in common. They called the conditions "risk factors," and they identified three primary risk factors and seven secondary risk factors for heart attack. The Framingham study was important for many reasons, but perhaps its most significant aspect had to do with the nature of the risk factors. Of the ten factors they identified, only three of them—all secondary—are beyond our control. The rest we can do something about.

The Seven Secondary Risk Factors

The word "secondary" here doesn't mean inconsequential; it simply means that these seven factors are less likely to lead to heart attack than the three primary ones, which we'll discuss in detail shortly. Each factor in both categories should be taken seriously in an assessment of your risks for heart disease.

HEREDITY

Heart disease runs in the family; it's as simple as that. Since there is nothing you can do about

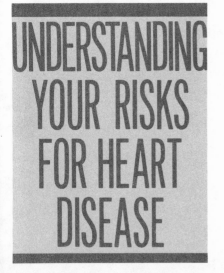

UNDERSTANDING YOUR RISKS FOR HEART DISEASE

your genes, if you fall into this high risk group, you have to be especially careful about avoiding the risk factors you can change. Maybe your parents have the disease because they smoke and drink and work 18-hour days, but that doesn't mean you have to do the same. Don't use them as role models for destructive behavior.

AGE

The older you are, the more likely you are to develop heart disease, probably (but not definitely) because you've had more years to drink, smoke, eat fatty foods, and suffer from tension. Again, the only way to deal with this factor is indirectly—by being especially strict about the others.

GENDER

Premenopausal women fall victim to heart disease less often than men, presumably because the extra estrogen produced by women prevents atherosclerosis. However, as women get older and produce less estrogen, they become as likely candidates for heart disease as men. It is possible that estrogen therapy for post-menopausal women helps to prevent heart disease, but the research is not conclusive.

STRESS

Some stress is unavoidable and even good for the health—many people feel that they can't perform well unless they're under stress—but too much stress, or the wrong kind, can raise your blood pressure and keep it up. Recognize the signs that you're suffering from too much of a good thing and learn how to control and combat those reactions with stress reduction techniques. (We mean relaxation exercises such as deep breathing, meditation, and yoga, not cocktails, cigarettes, and a quart of ice cream.) For more about stress and stress management techniques, see Chapters 16 and 17.

OBESITY

If you're obese, you probably know it, but just in case you don't, here's a medical definition. If you are a man, you are obese if you are more than 25 percent overweight. If you're a woman, it's more than 30 percent overweight. If you can get your weight down, you can lower your risk of heart disease. (You can also decrease your chances of developing diabetes, hypertension, and high cholesterol.) The best way to lose weight is slowly, through a combination of sensible eating and regular exercise.

INACTIVITY

Here's a quiz. Which single factor puts the greatest number of Americans in danger of developing heart disease? If you're like most people, your answer was hypertension, high cholesterol, or smoking. Wrong. According to the U.S. Center for Disease Control, the nation's most common cardiac threat is physical inactivity. Of course, it was sort of a trick question, since inactivity contributes to obesity, diabetes, high cholesterol, and hypertension. Moving your body on a regular basis can go a long way toward preventing heart disease.

DIABETES

Non-insulin dependent diabetes, sometimes called adult onset diabetes because it often strikes people over 40, is a double threat: first it's a disease in itself, caused by heredity, obesity, and inactivity; second it contributes to heart disease. Unlike juvenile (also called insulin-dependent) diabetes, adult onset is not typically treated with insulin, but it does respond to proper diet, weight loss, and exercise.

PRIMARY RISK FACTOR #1: HYPERTENSION

We're listing hypertension first of the three primary risk factors, but we could just as easily have started with high cholesterol or smoking. It's really too close a race to call. In this country some 60 million people suffer from hypertension. About 10 million take some sort of medication—to the tune of about $2.5 billion a year—but drugs notwithstanding, hypertension contributes to about 750,000 deaths every year. In addition to being a major cause of heart disease, hypertension (also called high blood pressure) is also the best-documented risk factor for stroke. About 70 percent of all stroke victims suffer from hypertension.

Hypertension is called the "silent killer," because it doesn't necessarily produce any noticeable symptoms. Unless you're starting to experience chest pains or shortness of breath, you may not even know you have it until you have a stroke, heart attack, or kidney failure.

WHO GETS IT?

Practically anyone can develop high blood pressure, but it's particularly prevalent among the middle-aged and elderly, obese people, blacks, heavy drinkers, women taking oral contraceptives, and people suffering from diabetes, gout, or kidney disease.

Some people have what's called "secondary" hypertension, which is caused by illness, such as diabetes or kidney disease. This kind is often curable. Many more hypertension sufferers—about 90 percent—have "essential" hypertension, which has no identifiable cause and no known cure. Of this group about 70 percent have only a mild case of hypertension, with a systolic blood pressure between 140 and 150 and diastolic between 90 and 104. Mild hypertension can get better, but it can also get worse.

WHAT CAUSES IT?

Time out for an anatomy lesson. The subject today is the circulatory system. Your body needs a constant supply of blood, to nourish it, aerate it, and remove waste products from it. The force that moves the blood comes from the heart, and the flow is regulated by a complex system of nerve signals, hormones, and other elements that widen or restrict the blood vessels (called arterioles). Your blood pressure depends on many factors, including the amount of blood flowing through the arteries, the rate of the flow, and the resiliency of the artery walls. When the arterioles are constricted for any reason, the pressure in the larger blood vessels rises. If it stays constricted, you end up with hypertension.

Hypertension causes atherosclerosis by injuring the artery walls and creating little cracks; the cracks collect cholesterol, which eventually develop into atherosclerotic plaques.

HOW TO PREVENT/CURE IT

Enough about what causes hypertension. Let's get on to a pleasanter and more productive subject: what you can do to avoid it or bring it under control. There are several areas in which you can make a real difference.

◆ Lose weight. Consider the following: (1) the incidence of hypertension among obese adults is estimated at double that of the non-obese; (2) studies of large population groups in countries where body weight does not generally increase with age indicate that blood pressure did not increase with age either (in America, land of the middle-age spread, about half the population has hypertension by 74 years old); and (3) hypertension sufferers who lost weight more than tripled their chances of safely discontinuing their blood pressure medication. There is no money-back guarantee that losing weight will lower your blood pressure, but it seems like a good bet. What's more, you don't have to lose a ton of weight to make a difference; a loss of even ten or so pounds over the course of a year can have a significant effect on bringing down your blood pressure, especially if your hypertension is mild.

◆ Exercise regularly. Aerobic exercise helps you control your weight and relieve stress, so you get a double whammy here.

◆ Cut down on your drinking. In Australia drinking beer is practically the national pastime, which makes it a good place to conduct a study. When the drinking habits of 20,000 Australians were examined, it was determined that the more they drank, the higher their blood pressure went. When age, obesity, and smoking were factored out, the role of alcohol became even more pronounced. In the United States alcohol consumption is blamed for about 10 percent of the hypertension in men.

♦ Learn to manage stress. Twenty-five percent of all sudden coronary deaths occur on Monday, and another 25 percent take place on Saturday. Why? The stress of sudden changes, as we wind up or wind down. Protect yourself by learning to control stress.

♦ Take medication. Since 1972, when the federal government launched a massive blood pressure awareness program, the heart disease rate has dropped by 34 percent, and the annual rate of fatal strokes has been cut dramatically. One important reason is blood pressure medication, especially beta blockers and diuretics. The news is not all good, though. The medicine can be expensive and side effects anything from mildly annoying to deeply disturbing. Some of the common ones are lethargy, constipation, hair loss, and impotence. Most doctors believe that non-drug treatments— diet, exercise, and stress management—are preferable to medication.

♦ Cut down on salt. Lowering your sodium intake often (but not always) brings blood pressure down. The American Heart Association says that no one should consume more than three grams of sodium a day and no more than 1000 milligrams (1 gram) for every 1000 calories. This involves more than throwing away the salt shaker; you also have to cut way back on packaged foods, read food labels closely, and learn what foods are naturally high in sodium.

♦ Avoid stimulants. Nicotine, caffeine, amphetamines, and diet pills have a tendency to raise blood pressure, at least temporarily. Although reports about their long-term effects on hypertension are inconclusive, it makes sense to use them sparingly, if at all, since they have other, better documented ill effects.

DOES ASPIRIN PREVENT HEART ATTACKS?

Maybe. Because aspirin prevents the accumulation of blood platelets, thereby reducing clot formation, one low-dosage aspirin, even baby aspirin, a day may reduce your risk of heart attack if you have coronary artery disease. (The benefits come from plain, buffered, or coated aspirin but not with acetaminophen or ibuprofen.) Aspirin therapy is not recommended for people with bleeding disorders, ulcers, diabetes, liver problems, or kidney disease or for anyone taking anti-coagulant drugs. Check with your doctor before you prescribe aspirin for yourself. And don't let swallowing an aspirin a day take the place of other, more significant behavior changes, such as losing weight, lowering cholesterol, and giving up cigarettes.

Primary Risk Factor #2: High Cholesterol

As we said earlier, we could very easily have listed high cholesterol as the number-one risk factor in heart disease, especially if it's not the only risk factor that applies to you. Cholesterol—the name given to blood fats, or lipids, in the body—is important in everyone, but if you smoke, if you have hypertension, or if you're diabetic, obese, or inactive, your cholesterol level becomes even more critical. According to the National Institutes of Health, about 5.4 million Americans need to lower their cholesterol. Many of them have no idea that they have a problem, since even if your cholesterol is dangerously high, you don't necessarily feel bad.

WHAT IS IT?

Here's another anatomy lesson. Coronary artery disease results when plaque accumulates on the walls of the arteries, blood flow is obstructed, and clots are formed. These clots may lead to a heart attack; often they do. The plaque that starts all the problems contains cholesterol. All blood contains some cholesterol. Your cholesterol count represents the number of milligrams of cholesterol per deciliter of blood.

Unlike many of the villains of good health, cholesterol is completely natural, essential to normal construction and function of the body. Contained in all cells in the body, cholesterol is especially prevalent in the organs; the heart, liver, brains, and kidneys have a high concentration of cholesterol. There's quite a bit in the adrenal glands and the sex glands as well, and cholesterol is a major component of the sex hormones.

Most of us are accustomed to thinking about cholesterol as something we eat, but that is not quite so. The body, specifically the liver, manufactures about two thirds of the cholesterol in the blood; naturally the amount produced that way is beyond your control. The remaining third of your cholesterol is dietary—related to what you eat—and that, of course, you can control.

HOW HIGH IS HIGH?

As of now the only way to determine your cholesterol level is with a blood test, and unfortunately all blood tests are not created equal; different labs may use different tests and consequently come up with different results. When you have the test done, be sure that the person doing it is trained in laboratory techniques and that the scale being used is the one provided by the national research group called the Lipid Research Clinics. The LRC's method is the most reliable, and if it's not the one your clinic uses, you may be comparing apples and oranges when you measure your progress.

There is continued debate about the recommended cholesterol level, with some of the loudest voices saying that anything over 180 is cause for some concern. In 1987, when the National Institutes of Health published their official guidelines, the cut-off was more like 200. Here are some of the other NIH standards.

AGE	NIH Standards for Cholesterol Levels	
	MODERATE RISK cholesterol greater than	HIGH RISK cholesterol greater than
2–19	170	185
20–29	200	220
30–39	220	240
40+	240	260

What this chart boils down to is this: if your cholesterol count is under 200, you can probably relax; just have it checked every few years. If you score between 200 and 239, you should modify your diet—cut your fats to 30 percent of your total diet, your saturated fats to 10 percent, and your cholesterol to 300 milligrams a day—and have your blood level checked once a year. If you're over 240, you should modify your diet and make a special effort to bring down your LDL cholesterol. If natural methods don't work within six months or so, drug therapy may be necessary.

It is generally accepted that the best overall indicator of cholesterol, especially for anyone over 50, is the ratio of your total cholesterol to your HDL or the ratio of HDL to LDL. For instance, if your total is 200 and your HDL is 50, the ratio is 4:1. The lower the number, the better off you are.

REVERSING THE DAMAGE

You can hardly pick up a newspaper or magazine today without reading something new, and probably contradictory to what you read last time, about cholesterol. The biggest news in a crowded field came in June 1987, when it was announced that the damage done by cholesterol is not necessarily permanent; reducing blood cholesterol will slow and in some cases reverse the build-up of artery-clogging plaque—good news for a change. Cholesterol can be lowered in any or all of several ways: diet, exercise, and medication. Let's take them one at a time.

LOWERING CHOLESTEROL THROUGH DIET Joe lives on pepperoni pizzas and cheese omelettes, and his cholesterol is 190. Sam, who gave up eggs in 1980 and has been following a low-fat diet religiously for the past two years, just found out that his is 210. What's going on? Is there no justice in the world? There may be justice in the world, but not when it comes to cholesterol. The fact of life is that people react to food in different ways. Some get fat while others stay thin; some can eat just one while others lose control; and some people are naturally blessed with low cholesterol despite a bad diet. That does not mean, however, that if your cholesterol is high, you should just throw your hands up in the air, curse Joe and all his kind, and accept your fate. Only a third of your cholesterol is dietary, but that third can prevent a heart attack. In Chapters 13 and 14 we discuss nutrition in full; that's where you'll find a more specific discussion of fats, carbohydrates, and fiber, for instance. Here we'll just make general recommendations.

♦ Decrease fats. Limit your total fat consumption to 20 percent of your total calories and your saturated fat to 10 percent. Cut down on red meat, whole milk dairy products, all kinds of oil, and processed foods.

♦ Decrease dietary cholesterol. Limit your cholesterol intake to 250 to 300 milligrams a day. (The American Heart Association recommends that you take in no more than 100 milligrams per 1000 calories). Since only animal products and by-products contain cholesterol in their natural form, that means being careful about anything in the milk and meat groups. Eggs and organ meats are the worst offenders in this category. An egg yolk has 255 milligrams of cholesterol (the white has none); 3.5 ounces of beef liver have 389 milligrams; the same amount of chicken liver logs in at 631.

♦ Increase fiber. Both kinds of fiber—soluble and insoluble—are good for your overall health, but soluble fiber actually lowers blood cholesterol by being absorbed into the bloodstream, latching on to the cholesterol, and literally pulling it out. The best sources for soluble fiber are oat products, especially oat bran, beans, legumes, and peas (dried or canned). The recommended daily ration is five to ten grams.

♦ Don't overdo protein. Because protein often doubles as a fat source, too much protein may mean way too much fat. Four to six ounces a day of protein are plenty, and the best sources are fish, skinless chicken and turkey, and lean cuts of pork, lamb, and beef.

♦ Make complex carbohydrates the staple of your diet. Sixty percent of your diet should come from complex carbohydrates: breads, cereals and grains, vegetables, and fruits. Be sure to choose the ones that are low in saturated fat and high in fiber; read the labels on cereal boxes, paying special attention to the fat content. Avoid biscuits, croissants, and muffins, except for the ones, packaged or home-baked, that are high in fiber and low in fat.

◆ Discover legumes and other meat substitutes. Kidney beans, lima beans, lentils, chickpeas, split peas, and other dried beans and peas are all excellent low-fat, high-fiber protein sources. Tofu is a good low-fat meat substitute. In many recipes egg whites may be used instead of whole eggs. Expand your horizons.

◆ Switch to low-fat dairy products. Try skim milk, low-fat cottage cheese and yogurt, and cheese made with vegetable oil. They may take a little getting used to, but as your cholesterol drops, you'll learn to love them.

◆ Increase your intake of fish oils. There is some evidence that Omega 3 fatty acids, the ones present in cold-water fish, can have a beneficial effect on your cholesterol level. The current wisdom is that eating three or four ounces of these oily fish (mackerel, tuna, and salmon, for instance) three or four times a week can lower your total cholesterol, raise your HDL, and lower your blood pressure. The only drawback is that these fish are relatively high in calories. It's some comfort to know that tuna packed in water works better than the more caloric kind packed in oil, because the Omega 3 tends to "leak out" into the oil.

LOWERING CHOLESTEROL THROUGH EXERCISE It would be nice to think that you could "burn up" cholesterol through exercise, the way you burn up fat, but it doesn't work that way. Cholesterol is not used as a fuel source in exercise. Still, exercise does have an indirect effect by producing hormones, which in turn affect the production of cholesterol.

Studies show that if you do 30 to 40 minutes of vigorous aerobic exercise (working at 70-80 percent of your maximal heart rate) four times a week, you can raise your HDL and lower your total cholesterol. This can't be a temporary program, though. It works only as long as you keep it up.

LOWERING CHOLESTEROL WITH DRUGS Diet and exercise are vastly preferable methods for lowering cholesterol, but sometimes the natural therapies just don't work. If after six months or so of working with diet and aerobic exercise you still have a dangerously high cholesterol level, your doctor will probably recommend medication. While drugs aren't usually the treatment of choice, they can be very effective in preventing heart attacks and even reversing the effects of cholesterol build-up. Some of the most commonly prescribed drugs are Questran, Lopid, and Mevacor. Drugs may lower cholesterol by anything from 10 to 50 percent, but there is a down side here. There is no such thing as a drug without a side effect; some of the ones associated with these are constipation, abdominal distress, blurred vision, muscle inflammation, and gastrointestinal problems.

THE TWO KINDS OF CHOLESTEROL

As we explained in Chapter 2, your total cholesterol count is broken down into two main parts: LDL and HDL. If they were starring in a western, LDL would wear the black hats and HDL would get white.

LDL, low-density lipoprotein, is light and fluffy. It meanders through the bloodstream, latches onto the tears in the arterial walls, and contributes to plaque build-up. Even more important than keeping your total cholesterol low is reducing your LDL, especially as you get older. The most effective ways of reducing LDL are dietary:

♦ Decrease your intake of saturated fats.
♦ Increase your consumption of monounsaturated fats.
♦ Raise the ratio of polyunsaturated fats to saturated fats in your diet.
♦ Decrease your caloric intake of all fats.
♦ Limit your daily protein intake to 4 to 6 ounces.
♦ Increase your intake of soluble fiber.
♦ Eat more foods high in Omega 3 fatty acids.
♦ Keep your weight under control. Lose weight if necessary.

A FEW WORDS ABOUT TRIGLYCERIDES

While we're on the subject of blood fats, we should probably spend a few moments talking about the other kind, triglycerides. The largest of the blood's oily particles, these lipids make up almost all of the blood fats known as the very low density lipoprotein, or VLDL.

There is less certainty among the medical establishment about whether elevated triglycerides are related to coronary artery disease. A low triglyceride count seems to be a sign of good health, but that may be coincidence; when triglycerides are low, so are blood pressure and cholesterol. The normal range is from 85 to 250 milligrams per deciliter of blood, and anything above 250 may be cause for concern.

Losing weight (even a few pounds), changing your diet, and getting regular exercise will usually bring your triglyceride level down.

Picture HDL, or high-density lipoprotein, as the police force of the bloodstream. It's the job of HDL to arrest the loitering LDL waiting to latch onto the arterial walls and cart them off to the liver. (To extend the metaphor even further, cops may turn bad when they drink; alcohol interferes with the action of HDL.) For obvious reasons, you want your HDL to be high; a higher number means a lower risk for heart disease. The optimal HDL level of the average woman is 65; for men it's 55. There are four ways to raise your HDL:

♦ Don't smoke.
♦ Stay active. Start a regular aerobic exercise program.
♦ Eat more soluble fiber.
♦ Eat more Omega 3 fatty acids.

PRIMARY RISK FACTOR #3: SMOKING

It's no secret that smoking is not just a bad habit. It's a menace to your health in general and to the heart and lungs in particular. It gives you lung cancer and heart disease, aggravates ulcers, and causes bronchitis and emphysema. It also causes birth defects, stillbirths, and low-weight babies, and it may be responsible for spontaneous abortions. It lowers your HDL cholesterol, and it brings on circulatory problems. In women it can also impair fertility and bring on early menopause. As if all that weren't enough, smoking doesn't help your looks either; many smokers have deep lines around their eyes and mouth and a grayish tinge to their skin.

It is estimated that one out of every seven deaths in the United States is smoking-related. The habit doubles the risk of heart attack and accounts for a third of all heart disease deaths. About 75 percent of emphysema deaths and 80 percent of all lung cancer deaths are caused by smoking. Smoking a pack of cigarettes a day decreases your life expectancy by six years; two packs a day rob you of about eight.

THE CHEMISTRY OF SMOKING

Smoke contains more than 4000 different compounds, not one of which is good for you. The worst offenders are arsenic, carbon monoxide, formaldehyde, nitrous oxide, hydrogen cyanide, and nicotine. Of those the one most hazardous to your health is nicotine, a colorless, poisonous alkaloid that is as addictive as heroin and just as dangerous. Within seven seconds after you inhale cigarette smoke, the nicotine in the smoke begins to stimulate the activity of neurochemicals in your body, which in turn affect your blood pressure, heart rate, blood sugar, and your sensitivity to pain. By first stimulating and then depressing the nervous system smoking also affects your mood, performance, and memory.

As you can imagine, all of this chemical activity plays havoc with the pulmonary system. Tar builds up in the lungs, and the lining of the nose and mouth becomes irritated. The short-term result is colds, flu, viruses, and other respiratory infections. In the long term it can result in lung cancer and emphysema. The cardiovascular system takes a terrible beating as well, with an increased heart rate, constricted arteries, irregular heartbeat, thickening of the arterial walls, and decreased oxygen supply. The most immediate results are poor circulation and hypertension.

Now that we have your attention, we'll cut to the chase. The only way to eliminate this risk factor from your life is to quit smoking. It's not the easiest thing in the world to do, but millions of people have tried and succeeded. All it takes is the knowledge of how to do it and a determination to succeed. We can help you with the first part, but only you can provide the second. If you're ready, do not pass Go or collect 200 dollars. Go directly to Chapter 23.

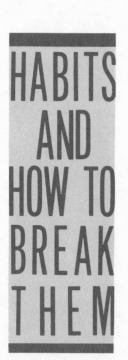

HABITS AND HOW TO BREAK THEM

4

We drink coffee until we get the jitters, nibble ourselves into obesity, drink too much alcohol, and ride when we can walk. We know that we should change our ways, but we can't—or, more accurately, we don't. If we're so smart, why aren't we perfect? Habit.

There are other reasons, too. For one, we're experts at denial. We refuse to believe that our actions have consequences, that if we smoke we'll get lung cancer or that having a bag of corn chips and a couple of beers every night is responsible for our high blood pressure. Another thing we're good at is rationalization. We tell ourselves that we need these cookies because we've been working so hard we didn't have time for dinner; or that we just don't have time to get on the exercise bike. We're also incredibly stubborn, sometimes clinging to our bad behavior as fiercely as if it were the Declaration of Independence. Whatever the reason for our undesirable behavior, many of us are heading for trouble if we don't change our ways.

Changing your behavior is easier said than done, no question about it, but it can and does happen. We see it every day at the Ranch, and for dozens of different reasons. Some guests make a change because they see the light. They finally understand that their actions have consequences. They realize, for instance, that they can lower their cholesterol level if they replace ice cream with frozen yogurt and corn chips with popcorn. Others get scared; they take a long look at their Health Risk Appraisals and understand for the first time that they're committing slow suicide. And then there are the ones who discover that all things considered, good habits just make you feel a whole lot better than bad ones.

We have found that many people who are highly

motivated when it comes to external things—making money, being successful in business, working on being a good spouse or parent—run out of steam when it comes to taking care of themselves. They readily accept the fact that business and social accomplishments require commitment and hard work, but somehow they can't apply that same kind of thinking to modifying their own behavior.

For everyone who wants to break a habit the first step is self-awareness, an understanding of what internal or external forces drive and motivate us. Is it guilt, fear, pride, vanity, a desire for approval or rewards, an inner voice? Which is more important, self-esteem or applause? Are you more likely to climb a mountain because it's there, because someone says he'll give you a thousand dollars if you make it to the top, or because you'll get your picture in the paper?

The key to motivation is desire. You have to want to reform, and you have to be honest about why. If the reasons aren't sound, you probably won't succeed. If you quit smoking because your kids have been nagging you, starve yourself to show off to your friends at a high school reunion, or go to a stress-reduction program because it's company policy, you're off to a bad start. If you do it for the right reasons, because you yourself want to live a longer, healthier, high-quality life, you're much more likely to make it.

If you've been to the beach, you've noticed that everyone has his own way of going into the water for the first time. Some people rush headlong into the waves; others get wet a toe at a time. People are like that with habits too. When it comes to changing habits, it pays to think long and hard about what you are about to do. Try the concept on for size. Picture yourself living with the new habits. Then choose a goal—realistic and preferably short-term—you can live with.

Once you've identified the goal, you still have some work to do. First you have to promise yourself that you'll do whatever it takes to reach it. If that means avoiding your friends until you've kicked the coffee habit, giving up TV because that's where you do your best nibbling, spending every night of your first week of non-smoking in a movie theater, or hiring a trainer to come in three times a week to supervise your workouts, so be it. If the only way you can keep from eating high-fat foods is to throw them out of the house, do it. Keep in mind that it took you a long time to form your bad habits, and it's going to take a while to break them.

No matter how determined you are and how strict, you may as well know in advance that you're probably going to have a slip or two. Remember, even though the behavior is bad it is an old friend; throwing out a bad habit can feel like casting off part of yourself. Even so, a setback can be discouraging, especially to highly motivated, successful people, who often have no concept of failure. Try not to beat yourself up. Failure can be educational; ask yourself why you fell back into your old ways and how you can keep it from happening again. Make sure the goals you set aren't beyond reach. Sometimes you have to fall a few times before you know how to stand on your feet.

The bottom line is this: anything you learn you can unlearn, as long as you want to do it and you have the correct tools for the job. The child in you may want to do what's familiar, to cling to the bad old ways, but the adult in you, the one who knows what's right for you, must take control and say, "Enough." Examine the patterns in your life. If you don't like what you see, choose a different pattern. Know that you can change, you can stop drinking or smoking or overeating or biting your nails or being inactive. But saying you've "got to" do something is not good enough. It's not what we have to do or need to do or should do or ought to do that governs our behavior. It's what we *want* to do.

THE 10 STEPS TO BREAKING A HABIT

There is a great deal of advice on breaking specific habits elsewhere in this book, especially in Parts II, III, and IV. Here are some general guidelines for changing behavior.

1   Understand your habitual responses. Be consciously aware that you have a habit. Notice, for example, that every time the phone rings, you automatically light up a cigarette or that whenever you hear the theme music of the nightly news, you crave a bowl of fudge ripple ice cream. Figure out how much of a habit you have—how "far gone" you are. If food is your problem, write down everything you eat. If you smoke, count your cigarettes. Keep track of the times you're most likely to be subject to stress. Figure out why you enjoy exercise on some days and dread it on others. If you can anticipate a habitual response, you are halfway toward getting rid of it.

2   Make your goals specific. Saying that you're going to start "eating right" or "getting some exercise" or that you "have to learn to relax" won't do it. The only way you can reach a goal is to know precisely what it is: eating only at mealtimes, hitting the rowing machine for a half-hour four times a week, having a glass of water and taking a deep breath every hour on the hour, or anything else.

3   Visualize yourself without the bad habit. Picture yourself knitting instead of smoking, reading a magazine instead of chowing down on potato chips, or sitting up straight at your desk instead of slouching. If you have a business trip coming up, get a mental picture of yourself doing laps in the hotel pool every morning and having fruit for dessert every night.

4   Develop a support system. Tell your family and friends and co-workers what you're up to. Try to get others to join you; it probably wouldn't hurt everyone in your office to stop drinking coffee, for instance. Don't be ashamed to ask for a pep talk when you're down or a standing ovation when you've got good news. You need all the help you can get.

5   Reevaluate your goals regularly. We all make mistakes; you may have made one when you set your original goal. Maybe running 10 miles a day seven days a week, rain or shine, was a little too much to ask of yourself. Perhaps life without a speck of chocolate is not working out. Every week or so take time out for a reality check. How are you doing? Is it working? If not, don't throw the whole plan out; just modify it. Try running three miles a day five days a week and fitting a small piece of chocolate into your meal plan.

6   Pamper yourself a little. Saying goodbye to an old friend can be tough, so you'd be wise to make it up to yourself in other, nondestructive ways. If you have a full day, schedule time to unwind, even if it's only a few minutes to get up and stretch and walk around the room. Set aside 10 minutes to meditate. Better yet, leave work an hour early and get a massage or go for a walk in the park.

7   Reward yourself often. Don't wait until you've reached your ultimate goal to give yourself a pat on the back for a job well done. Do it early and often. Take in a play you've been wanting to see, have a massage, get a facial, sleep late, take a vacation, buy a piece of jewelry or a new set of golf clubs, go to a ball game. If you forget about rewards, you are more likely to backslide.

8   Be on the lookout for self-sabotage. Strangely enough, the closer you get to your goal, the more likely you are to return to your old behavior. If you feel your resolve weakening, remind yourself of your original goals and redouble your efforts. Focus on the present, not on how far you've come.

9   Accept an occasional slip. If you do get off the track, keep your "failure" in perspective. If you're driving home from work and have a craving for an ice cream cone, ask yourself if something else will do the trick. Maybe an apple or a banana or a new magazine will satisfy that craving. Think before you act. If you do end up having the ice cream, give yourself permission to enjoy it and then get on with it. Don't dwell on past defeats.

10 Keep a sense of humor. When you want a cigarette or a brownie so badly you could scream, you may not feel like smiling, but give it a try. It helps.

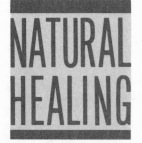

5

NATURAL
HEALING

The title on the door to Dr. Andrew Weil's office says "Natural Healing," but it might just as well say "Last Resort." Many of the guests who end up in his office have been everywhere and tried everything. The only problem is, they're still sick.

"Six months ago I saw a woman who had been quite seriously ill for 12 years," said Andrew. "It all started with a urinary dysfunction. She consulted several doctors, but no one could come up with an explanation for what was bothering her. She took antibiotics, but they didn't help. She saw another set of doctors, but they didn't have any luck either. A couple of them said her condition was all in her mind. She stayed with the antibiotics, but after several years of not feeling better she started feeling worse. The urinary dysfunction was still there, and now she'd developed pain during intercourse. That meant more doctors, one of whom recommended reconstructive surgery. The surgery didn't help, though; the pain was still there. The physical problems and the stress they brought on caused her marriage to break up.

"When she came to see me, she was pretty much at the end of her rope. In 12 years she had seen 20 physicians, and she felt worse that day than ever. We spent a couple of hours going over her health history, and one of the hundreds of things she told me was that although she loved to drink coffee, she could drink only two cups a day; if she drank more, her hands would start to shake. I suspected that she was addicted to caffeine, and I told her to kick the habit. I warned her that she might have a rough time of it, and she did. For three or four days she went through severe withdrawal symptoms, but some of the herbal remedies, breathing techniques, and visualization I taught her helped her get through it. Within a week she started to feel better. Within four months all her urinary complaints disappeared, and her anxiety level dropped 90 percent. She hadn't needed surgery or antibiotics. She just needed to stop drinking coffee."

Another, equally distraught woman here at the Ranch complained to Andrew about being tired all the time. She had no energy at all, and she couldn't seem to digest her food properly. There were a dozen other unpleasant symptoms, none of which she could understand or explain. The woman had seen a half-dozen doctors, but none of them could cure what ailed her. Most of the doctors thought that her problem was emotional (the woman had a high-pressure job and traveled a great deal) and recommended psychotherapy. However, what Andrew discovered the woman really needed was medicine—specifically, medication to treat an underactive thyroid. After a few weeks of taking her newly prescribed medicine the woman was the picture of health.

We tell these two stories to make a simple point: there is no "right" system of medicine. Every system cures some of the people some of the time, even when its methods are as far "wrong" as science can go. No system has a monopoly on failure, either. Every system *doesn't* work some of the time too, including orthodox medicine. One person can be cured by withdrawing from caffeine; with another the miracle comes in the shape of a thyroid pill. The right medicine is the one that works. And a philosophical prejudice in favor of one approach over another may keep the patient from his best cure.

You Take Charge

The basic difference between orthodox medicine, called allopathy, and natural healing therapies is that there is a level of participation and awareness in natural healing that is not necessary in allopathy. After all, you don't have to "participate with" your antibiotics; you just have to take them as many times a day as it says on the label. In natural healing you not only are involved 100 percent in the healing process; you are the one in charge.

Most of us assume that healing is something that is done to us, just as we assume that pain and illness are imposed on us, yet we aren't strangers to the self-healing process. When we cut ourselves, the bleeding stops, and the skin knits back together. When we have surgery, the doctor sews us up, but we take it from there. Every human being is born with the ability to heal himself. We also have a natural resistance to illness, at least most of the time. Notice that you don't always get an allergic reaction just because you meet an allergen, and you don't always have to get an infection just because you come into contact with germs.

In the past many people thought of natural healing as a radical or mystical alternative to conservative medical care. Today millions say that alternatives to standard medical care—particularly in the treatment of asthma, ulcers, allergies, heart disease, cancer, lupus, and arthritis—are a must.

What Is Natural Healing?

Think of your body as a big pot filled with water. When you get sick, a fire is lit under the pot, the water boils, and steam begins to rise from the pot. Obviously the best way to stop the steam is to put out the fire, but what we do instead is put a lid on the pot. That's the biggest problem with scientific medicine: it's suppressive in nature, not curative. By putting a lid on the steaming pot allopathic medicine suppresses the symptoms instead of curing the disease. Natural healing recognizes that the human body is equipped to resist disease and heal injuries—to put out the fire under the pot.

To understand the power of natural healing you must begin to look at health and disease in new ways. Our natural inclination, when we're sick or injured, is to see if there is something invasive that will make us feel better: a pill, a splint, or an operation, for instance. By definition natural healing therapies are those that are non-invasive; they don't involve chemotherapy, surgery, radiation, or any of the other therapies in the allopathic tool bag. Natural healing has its own tools, however. Among the ones we rely on most heavily at the Ranch—in addition to exercise and a sensible diet—are meditation, breathing techniques, herbal treatments, massage, hypnotherapy, biofeedback, and MindFitness. Other tried-and-true natural healing remedies are naturopathy, homeopathy, osteopathic manipulative treatment, and acupuncture. (See Chapters 17, 19, and 20 for more about stress management techniques, herbal therapies, and massage.)

Treating Addictive Behavior

Most of us develop some kind of addictive behavior in order to calm ourselves. The majority of people who need to relax use either drugs, by which we mean caffeine, nicotine, and alcohol as well as over-the-counter and prescription (or even illegal) drugs, or food. When we get frazzled, some of us reach for cigarettes or a dry martini; others of us turn to doughnuts or pepperoni pizza.

The nicotine in cigarettes is by far the most addictive drug around. Alcohol is one of the strongest and most toxic of all drugs, although some people are perfectly capable of using alcohol non-addictively. Caffeine is a very strong drug, with a high potential for addiction. Most coffee drinkers are addicted to caffeine, but unlike the woman whose story we told at the beginning of this chapter, the majority are not debilitated by the addiction. (For more about caffeine and alcohol see Chapters 13 and 14.) The most common addiction, and perhaps the hardest to deal with, is food addiction. By that we mean not eating disorders such as bulimia or anorexia but rather an overall difficulty in limiting the intake of food.

Natural healing therapies are an essential part of learning to put an end to addictive behavior of any kind. The first step is to look at the behavior and ask yourself what you can do to encourage your body to heal itself. You have to find those systems that allow you to find the "on" switch that gives you the power to change. The systems will be different for everyone—breathing, massage, hypnotherapy, herbal treatments, yoga, meditation, or all of the above—but the process of finding the key is the same.

Treating Stress

Regardless of what causes an illness, it is unquestionably aggravated by stress, so one of the most important aspects of natural healing is stress management. (The various techniques are explained and examined in Chapter 17.) Almost everyone who sees Andrew Weil learns breathing exercises, and many are encouraged to try hypnotherapy, meditation, yoga, and biofeedback as well. Sometimes he tells his patients not to exercise quite so much.

As Andrew explains it, "One of the questions I ask my patients is, 'What do you do to relax?' If a person's answer is exercise, that indicates trouble to me. The reason is this. Exercise is a way of dealing with tension, but it does so just by burning it up. Exercise is fine—in fact, it's a lot better than fine—but it doesn't take the place of relaxation techniques that get to the root of the problem. Exercise treats symptoms, by getting you to stop grinding your teeth, for instance, or tiring you out so that you can sleep better. It does not get to what is causing the stress."

Healing with Herbs

When Great-Grandma's baby had a chest cold, she treated it the old-fashioned way, with eucalyptus vapor, white willow bark tea, perhaps a little Tiger Balm on the infant's chest. As anyone who has ever soothed an agitated stomach with a cup of peppermint tea knows, Great-Grandma knew what she was doing. There was and is a natural sympathy between herbs, plants, vegetables—anything that grows—and the human body. One of the most important elements of natural healing is the therapeutic use of herbs and medicinal plants.

Generally speaking, herbs are better for the body than more unnatural and unfamiliar synthetics—every known prescription and over-the-counter drug has side effects, many of them quite undesirable—but that does not mean that any herb or plant will do. There are three basic types of herbs: the beverage herbs, such as spearmint, peppermint, and chamomile, which may be consumed in large quantity without ill effects; the medicinal herbs, which are stronger and more powerful and should be used under the supervision of an herbalist, a pharmacologist, or some other expert; and the dangerous herbs, which should be avoided. Some herbs are poisonous, with undesirable side effects ranging from mild nausea to serious cardiovascular or nervous system damage. Herbs in this third category include arnica, belladonna, bittersweet twigs, hemlock, heliotrope, calamus, bloodroot, broom-top, henbane, jalap root, jimson weed, lobelia, lily of the valley, mandrake, mistletoe, morning glory, periwinkle, St. Johnswort, spindle-tree, tonka bean, wahoo bark, worm-wood, white snakeroot, and yohimbi. None of these dangerous herbs will be for sale in health food stores.

Try the following, perfectly safe herbal remedies for common maladies:

♦ For a cold. Rub some Tiger Balm on your chest and below each nostril and take an herbal bath with a mixture of eucalyptus, chamomile, and spearmint. To prepare the bath tie three ounces of each of the three herbs in a muslin or cheesecloth bag or a cotton T-shirt. Fill the tub half full with very hot water and let the herb mixture steep for about eight minutes, squeezing the bag occasionally. Add enough cool or warm water to make the bath comfortable and enjoy a long soak.

♦ For fever. The best thing for fever is to sweat it out. One good way is to take a steaming hot shower, closing the door and letting the bathroom get really hot. After spending a few minutes taking the hottest shower you can stand, wrap up in a robe, cover your head with a towel, and sit in the still-steaming bathroom under three or four layers of wool blankets. Sweat it out for 15 or 20 minutes, then start taking off the layers and cooling down gradually. When you're comfortable, dry off with a towel, change into a warm flannel nightshirt, and crawl into a nice warm bed.

♦ For congestion. The last thing at night and first thing in the morning inhale eucalyptus vapor. To six quarts of boiling water add an ounce of eucalyptus leaves and let them steep for eight minutes. Put your head over the pot (not so close that you get scalded, of course) and cover your head and the pot with a large towel. Inhale through your nose and exhale through your mouth for five minutes; then inhale through your mouth and exhale through your nose for five minutes. If you like, you can also strain the leaves and put the liquid into a vaporizer near your bed.

♦ For a sore throat or swollen glands. Gargle with salt water (a tablespoon of sea salt in 12 ounces of very warm water); massage oil of peppermint into your throat; and suck on natural herbal throat lozenges or chew on a licorice root stick. Other cough drops and lozenges are full of sugar and sometimes alcohol, which just weaken your system further.

The Non-Medicine Cabinet

Take a long, hard look in your medicine cabinet. If you're like most people, you'll find a veritable pharmacy in there—sleeping pills, laxatives, antacids, eye drops, nasal sprays, antihistamines, aspirin, mouthwash. For many of the jars and bottles in your cabinet there's a natural remedy that may be used as a substitute. Most are available at health food stores or through mail order companies. (One good one is Eclectic Institute, Inc., 11231 SE Market Street, Portland, Oregon 97202.) If you'd like to give herbal remedies a try, here are some places to start.*

INSTEAD OF THIS	TRY THIS	IN THIS FORM
ASPIRIN	white willow bark	Steep 1 tsp. in a cup of boiling water for 3 to 5 minutes. Drink.
TRANQUILIZERS	chamomile (mild) or valerian (strong)	Steep 1 tsp. in a cup of boiling water for 10 minutes. Drink.
ANTACIDS	spearmint or peppermint	Steep 1 tsp. in a cup of boiling water for 3 to 5 minutes. Drink.
LAXATIVES	senna	Steep 2 gelatin capsules of the herb in 2 cups boiling water for 15 minutes. Cool and drink.
CAFFEINE	ginseng or licorice root	Chew a piece of the root.
FIRST-AID CREAMS	aloe vera	Cut open a stalk from the plant. Squeeze gel onto burn.
DECONGESTANTS	eucalyptus	Steep 1 oz. in 6 qts. boiling water for 10 minutes. Cover head with a towel and breathe in until congestion clears or strain and pour into a vaporizer.
NASAL SPRAY	Tiger Balm ointment (white is mild; red is strong)	Place a tiny amount below each nostril.
EYE-WHITENER DROPS	golden seal	Steep 1 tsp. in 4 oz. boiling water until it's completely cool. Drop in your eye with an eye dropper.
INSECT REPELLENT	citronella oil	Rub onto skin.
BREATH FRESHENER	parsley	Chew a fresh sprig.

* Chart courtesy of *Mademoiselle* magazine, August 1986.

TREATING DISEASE

One sunny December afternoon Deborah Morris, another natural healing practitioner at the Ranch, began one of her attitudinal healing lectures by telling the story of a good friend of hers who died suddenly, after a ten-day bout with cancer. At 40 years old her friend was totally unprepared to die. Hopeless and helpless, he lacked the resources to cope with his impending death. In some ways the saddest part of the story, according to Morris, is that he didn't get a chance to learn anything from his disease.

Not surprisingly, some of the people listening to this story became a little uncomfortable. After all, who wants to talk about death and disease? They're depressing subjects, and besides, it's morbid to dwell on things like that. We're meant to be thinking about being well!

Deborah Morris doesn't think it's morbid or depressing to think about sickness; she thinks it's essential. She also thinks that people don't get sick arbitrarily. It's not just happenstance that brings illnesses into people's lives. Illnesses are opportunities, which take you on a particular path to making changes. No matter how careful we all are, virtually all of us will be sick at least once before we die, and when that happens, we will have a choice: we can feel sorry for ourselves; we can medicate ourselves; or we can change our behavior and get on with our lives. Our attitude about our illnesses affects our ability to cope with them. The time to prepare for sickness and become familiar with the tools that help us feel better is when we are healthy and well.

KEEPING AN OPEN MIND

In one form of Zen meditation there is a kind of policeman on duty. He carries a stick and walks up and down the rows of assembled meditators, keeping an eye on them. If he notices that someone's posture is poor or that his concentration is beginning to waver, he walks up behind the "slacker" and hits him sharply with the stick. This seemingly cruel and unusual punishment has given rise to many stories of instant enlightenment: apparently being hit with a stick was exactly what some people needed to wake them up.

At Canyon Ranch there are no sticks, but we do try to wake people up. We give our guests the tools and techniques that will let them feel better, whether that means the ability to prevent an asthma attack or the power to resist a chocolate chip cookie, a cigarette, or a drink. Maybe the next time they have a headache, they'll have something they can do about it

HOW TO FIND A NATURAL HEALING THERAPIST

Deciding to explore the possibilities of natural healing therapies is only the first step. Next you must decide which therapy—and therapist—is best for you. In any sort of healing process, belief in the treatment is crucial. The practitioner must believe in what he or she is doing, and the patient must believe that it will work. Natural healing will only do you good if the theories become yours.

First look for licensed medical doctors who are open-minded about alternative medicine. (The American Holistic Medical Association, at 2002 East Lake Avenue East, Seattle, Washington 98102, will give you a list of holistic practitioners in your part of the world.) Ask your own doctors if they prescribe natural healing therapies. When you're interviewing potential therapists, don't be afraid to ask the hard questions: Where were you trained? How long did the training last? Where have you worked before? May I see your references? The therapist should be willing to answer all of your questions directly; if he's reluctant to do so, try someone else. Be careful of anyone who makes a diagnosis or prescribes medication or who says he or she can cure you. The person you're looking for is someone who will teach you, guide you, and provide encouragement, not somebody who promises miracle cures.

besides take two aspirin. Whatever the problems are that they're fighting—five extra pounds or a drinking problem or a crazy boss—they no longer feel helpless and hopeless in dealing with them.

We're not suggesting that you stop seeing doctors or throw away your medicine. We're only saying that you need to begin to open yourself up to new things that might work. Don't let skepticism or a fear of the unknown prevent you from trying something new. Breakthroughs come from breaking down barriers. You owe it to yourself to keep an open mind, to look at the way you're living and to make changes based on what you see so that you can reduce your chances of getting sick.

We know more than any culture has ever known before about how to be healthy and well, yet we are not anywhere near being able to achieve what we know. Where is the gap between what we know and what we do? The gap lies within us. Real inspiration is allowing people to use what they already know.

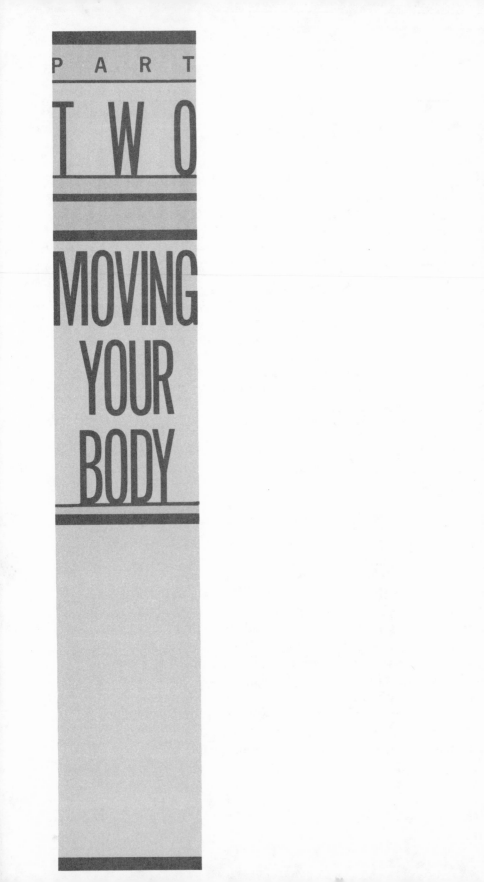

PART
TWO

MOVING
YOUR
BODY

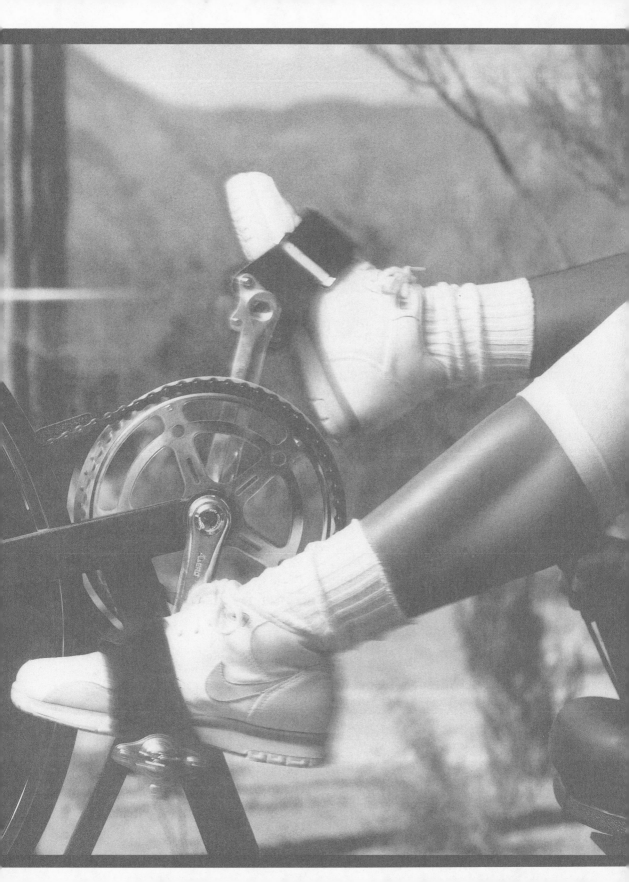

6

At Canyon Ranch our guests make remarkable discoveries every day. They find out, for instance, that they can live without caffeine, that herbal wraps and massages are as soothing and relaxing as everyone says, and that a small bag of unsalted popcorn can taste pretty darned good when it's all you have. Perhaps the most important overall discovery that our guests make during their stay is that it feels great to move their bodies. Many come here already knowing that exercise is good for them, but others haven't broken a sweat or breathed hard with exertion in years, let alone worked on their calf muscles or flexed their pecs. It doesn't take novices very long to understand that exercise is the cornerstone of our program.

With every passing day the medical message becomes clearer: the key component in wellness is exercise. If you don't move your body, you're going to pay the price.

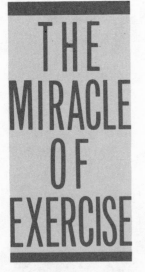

THE MIRACLE OF EXERCISE

WHAT EXERCISE DOES

At the Ranch we find that once people understand something about the physiology of exercise—about the specific benefits of working up a sweat and getting out of breath on a regular basis—they are more likely to embrace it. Sometimes it's enough just to say that active people live anywhere from 11 to 15 percent longer than sedentary people, not to mention the fact that the quality of those extra years is likely to be a lot better too. For those who need more, here are a few of the more specific benefits.

YOUR CARDIOVASCULAR SYSTEM

As you get older and move around less, your body gradually loses its ability to deliver and use oxygen as a fuel source—on the average the loss in capacity is .5 to 1 percent per year from age 30 on. You're not likely to notice much of a change until middle age, but by age 50 the difference is often quite apparent; all of a sudden you just can't do as much as you used to. The simple fact is that while some decline is natural and unavoidable, sedentary people decline much more rapidly than those who remain active. The more you exercise, the stronger you will remain.

Recent studies conducted by the Stanford Center for Research in Disease Prevention concluded that people who burned 2000 calories a week in moderate exercise significantly improved their cardiovascular fitness as well as reducing weight and body fat.

YOUR WEIGHT

Everyone accepts the fact that eating less makes you lose weight. Only relatively recently have people begun to appreciate that exercise is just as important to weight control as counting calories, perhaps even more. In addition to burning calories exercise raises your metabolic rate, and it may play a part in suppressing appetite. Certainly it increases your awareness of your body, which often makes it easier for you to control your eating; once you know that it takes 20 minutes of running to "work off" one chocolate chip cookie, it becomes harder to eat 5 or 6 or 20 at a sitting. All the dietitians in the world won't make or keep you fit and keep the pounds off. You have to move your body.

YOUR MUSCLES AND BONES

If someone breaks his arm and has to wear a cast for six weeks, by the time the cast comes off, the muscles in his arm will have shrunk a little and become stiff. If you don't exercise regularly, it's as if you're in a total body cast; you atrophy and stiffen. Studies indicate that a patient confined to his bed loses up to 8 grams of muscle mass a day and about 1½ grams of calcium a week from the bones. With a regular regimen of weight-bearing activities or strength training you can keep your bones and muscles flexible and strong.

YOUR MOOD

This is trickier to measure than blood pressure or body fat. How do you calculate inner peace, self-esteem, or a general sense of well-being? How can you prove that exercise decreases stress and anxiety? It's not easy. We do know that when a person exercises vigorously, morphine-like substances called endorphins are released into the bloodstream, and these are responsible for producing an enhanced feeling of well-being. We also know that people are happier when they exercise than when they don't. Regular exercise does wonders for your attitude toward every aspect of your life.

THE COMPONENTS OF FITNESS

The three components of fitness are cardiovascular endurance, flexibility, and muscular strength/endurance. Cardiovascular endurance is the body's maximum ability to take in, transport, and utilize oxygen; flexibility is the range of motion about a joint; and muscular strength/endurance is the ability of a muscle group to exert force and maintain a degree of force over a period of time.

Since all of these elements are necessary for fitness (we deal with each separately, in Chapters 7, 8, and 9), we are reluctant to rank them, but the fact is that the most important of the exercises are the ones that challenge the cardiovascular system: aerobic exercises, such as walking, running, swimming, cycling, hiking, rowing, cross-country skiing, jumping rope, and aerobic dance. Any aerobic activity will do, provided it satisfies a few qualifications:

♦ Frequency of activity. Opinions vary about how often you must have an aerobic workout to keep your heart healthy. Most experts say that three days a week is the minimum; others recommend four days a week for minimal cardiovascular endurance. For weight loss you'll probably need to work out five days a week.

♦ Duration of activity. Again, estimates vary, but the general guidelines call for exercising long enough to burn about 300 calories, which can mean anything from 20 to 40 minutes of continuous high-intensity activity. (In Chapter 7 there is a chart that gives the calorie-burning value of most aerobic exercises.) Intermittently intense activities, such as tennis or racquetball, may take up to 90 minutes or even longer to fill the calorie requirements.

♦ Intensity of activity. Walking a few blocks to the store is better than driving, and working in the garden is better than watching television, but neither of them counts as aerobic exercise, because that kind of activity doesn't raise your heart rate sufficiently or make you use enough oxygen. It's very simple, really: if you don't work hard enough, the exercise doesn't do what it's supposed to do.

WARMING UP, COOLING DOWN

No matter what your exercise of choice is, in order to exercise efficiently and avoid injuries it's vitally important to spend a little time warming up before you get going and cooling down when you're through. Easy, slow movement—a five-minute walk before a run, some easy stretches before you hop on the exercise bike, even a little limbering up before you get into the pool—prepares the muscles, joints, tendons, heart, and lungs for what's coming next.

An equally important part of any exercise regimen is the cool-down period. During exercise you make your heart and muscles work overtime, and there's a lot of extra blood pumping through your veins. When you stop exercising abruptly, the sudden drop in blood pressure may cause nausea, indigestion, light-headedness, hypothermia, and muscle weakness. The best cooling down exercise is a slow-motion version of what you have been doing: runners should jog and then walk; swimmers should switch to an easy stroke; cyclists should stay off hills and take it slow. Then take a few extra minutes to stretch out your thoroughly warm muscles. (See Chapter 8.) Wait until your heartbeat is down to 120 beats per minute before you hit the showers.

WHEN TO EXERCISE

Everyone has a theory. Some say that it's best to exercise late in the day because the metabolic jolt you get may keep you from overeating at night, which is what most people do. Others say an early morning workout keeps the metabolism up when it can do the most good, while you're awake. The problem with theories is that they have nothing to do with two important realities: first, we all have natural body rhythms (some of us just can't get moving in the morning, for instance, and others completely run out of steam by six o'clock); and second, we all have schedules. Don't worry about theories; the best time to exercise is when you want to and when you can.

FOOD AND EXERCISE

It's five o'clock, and you're on your way to the gym for your workout. It's been a long time since lunch, and your stomach is starting to growl; your blood sugar is low, and you're feeling a little weary. You can't decide whether to eat something. On the one hand, you don't want to feel weighed down when you hit the rowing machine; on the other hand, you're so hungry you're not sure you can make it.

Or maybe you like to run four miles first thing in the morning. If you have breakfast, you cramp up some time around mile two, but if you go out empty, your energy level is pathetic.

What are you supposed to do about food?

For some people, especially those with cast-iron stomachs, the food-exercise dilemma doesn't create much of a problem. In fact, only triath-aloners and other serious athletes really need to worry about it. Still, it's a good idea to understand how the body works so that you can make a judgment about the best way to fuel it.

When you exercise vigorously, your muscles need 75 to 85 percent of your body's blood for fuel. However, when you eat, the flow of blood is diverted to your stomach, where it aids digestion. If you exercise too soon after eating, the blood will still be in the stomach, unavailable to fuel the muscles. Without that blood the muscles will tire much more quickly. That's why it's a good idea not to eat anything for about two hours before a vigorous workout.

When you do need something to satisfy your hunger and keep you going through a workout, choose complex carbohydrates. Protein and fat linger too long in the stomach, diverting energy for digestion away from the muscles, and simple sugars, such as candy, cakes, and cookies, make your blood sugar soar and then drop, leaving you drowsy and definitely not in the mood for jumping rope. Rice cakes, whole wheat crackers, or an apple may not make your mouth water as much as a chocolate bar or a jelly doughnut, but they'll carry you through much better. The perfect pre-jog breakfast is a small meal (300 calories or fewer) high in carbohydrates with no sugar and no fat: for instance, oatmeal, cereal with skim milk, a piece of plain toast, or a piece of fruit.

It's a good idea to have a rice cake, a piece of bread, some fruit juice, low-fat yogurt, or an apple close at hand when you've finished your workout; although exercise suppresses some people's appetites, if only temporarily, others become ravenous the moment they stop moving. Glycogen (found in carbohydrates) makes the body run, and the stores of glycogen used up in vigorous exercise must be replenished fairly soon. Remember too that the body needs to be cooled and hydrated after exercise; nothing does that better than drinking lots of water.

GETTING STARTED

The best thing about the human body is that it's incredibly resilient. No matter how old you are, or how overweight and out of condition, you can make a change. The law of supply and demand in exercise is this: when you increase the demand for energy, the supply will be there. It may take you a while to reach your goal, but you'll get there. It's never too late to bring the "dead" back to life.

You're probably going to be discovering muscles you've long since forgotten and making demands on yourself that you haven't made in years, but don't be discouraged. Remember, even moderate exercise is better than none. A little yard work or home repairs, an evening of ballroom dancing, a half-mile stroll to pick up the morning papers, or walking up a couple of flights of stairs once or twice a day—it's all good stuff. The important thing is to get moving.

EXERCISE'S GREATEST MYTHS

Myth #1: You can spot-reduce. No, you can't. You can burn fat (through aerobic exercise), but you can't trim it from specific places on your body. Sit-ups and leg lifts increase your muscular endurance, but they don't get rid of spare tires, cellulite, or saddlebags.

Myth #2: No pain, no gain. That slogan has been replaced by, "Train, don't strain." There is nothing wrong with pushing yourself a little; meeting a challenge offers many physical and emotional satisfactions. But exercise does not have to feel bad to do you good.

Myth #3: You shouldn't exercise every day. Many people insist on a day of rest every week, but there's no physical reason not to do *some* kind of exercise every day if your body feels good and you want to do it. (As you'll see in Chapter 9, you shouldn't lift weights two days in a row.)

Myth #4: Exercising for more than 40 minutes is a waste of time. While the cardiovascular requirements of fitness are satisfied by anywhere from 20 to 40 minutes of high-intensity work, there are plenty of benefits of a longer workout. It increases endurance, burns more calories, and it can feel great.

Myth #5: Working at more than 85 percent of your maximal heart rate is dangerous. It's not necessarily dangerous—in fact, if you feel all right, it's perfectly acceptable—but we recommend against it anyway. As you'll see in Chapter 7, working somewhere between 60 and 85 percent of capacity gives you an excellent aerobic workout. Think of yourself as a finely tuned, efficient-running automobile. When you're working at more than 85 percent of your capacity, you're revving your engine.

Myth #6: You can't teach an old dog new tricks. It's true that everyone's body is not designed for gymnastics, marathon running, or competitive swimming, but it's also true that everyone, regardless of body type or fitness level, can retrain his muscles and make himself stronger, more flexible, and more aerobically fit. The only way to do that, however, is (you guessed it) by moving your body on a regular basis. Anything your body can learn it can unlearn.

STICKING TO YOUR PROGRAM

At Canyon Ranch we move all the time. Guests, even normally sedentary ones, think nothing of an action-packed day that takes them from a four-mile walk at seven in the morning to a rousing game of Wallyball at five in the evening, with a half-dozen classes in between and a quick half-hour on the treadmill before bed. Surrounded as they are with good choices, they start to think about their bodies in a new way. When they hear us preach the gospel of exercise, they nod their heads and vow that, of course, they'll take time every day to exercise, or at least five days a week.

But then they go back to the Real World, where they have a lot more on their minds, not to mention their schedules, than deciding between Stretch and Flex and Low-Impact Aerobics. How do they, and those of you who haven't been to the Ranch, get and stay motivated to stick to a sensible exercise program? Here are ten suggestions.

1   Examine your motives. Ask yourself exactly what you are trying to accomplish with your exercise program. Do you want to lose weight, lower your blood pressure, ease stress, reshape your body, be more flexible, improve your tennis game, lower blood pressure, control your diabetes, or all of the above? Are you frustrated with how you feel or how you look or both? Or are you just doing all this so that your doctor and/or family will quit nagging you? Before you can make a real commitment to changing your behavior, you have to understand why you're doing it.

2   Set reasonable goals. Make sure that what you want from an exercise program is, in fact, achievable. Set goals that can be met in a short period of time—two or three weeks at the most. A weight-loss goal of 25 pounds may take too long to reach; you'll be much happier if you take it five pounds at a time. Be realistic about exercise and weight loss. Exercising vigorously for a half hour burns about 300 calories; that means you have to work out for more than five hours to burn off one pound.

3   Choose the right activity. The only "wrong" exercise for you is the one you don't do. The fitness activity you pick has to suit your personality, your health needs, your schedule, and your tastes, not to mention the weather conditions in your part of the world. Figure out exactly where you can and will be able to make changes in your behavior. Think about your average day: what time you get up, when you have your meals, whether you're tired at the end of the work day or ready for action. Think about whether you're the solitary, self-motivating type (in which case you may like walking, running, or swimming) or the kind who needs company, supervision, or maybe even policing

and competition (squash, racquetball, aerobics classes). If you're
going to join a gym, find one that's convenient; a club membership
won't do you any good if the health club is closed when you're ready
for your workout. Most importantly, think about what you enjoy
doing. Fitness is supposed to be fun.

4   Be flexible. It's all very well to find an exercise you love, but what are
you supposed to do when it's snowing outside, the gym is closed, your
squash partner is busy, and your hamstrings are sore? You're supposed
to do something else. Switching can be difficult—people who love their
exercise bikes don't usually like to jog or jump rope, and most runners
would rather fight than swim—but a change of pace is a good idea once
in a while. It lets you work out different muscle groups, and it keeps
you from getting bored with your regular workout. When you pick an
alternate exercise regimen, try to choose something that travels well.

5   Be consistent. One of the most critical elements of any exercise
program is consistency, but the most overused excuse in the book for
skipping exercise is, "I don't have time." Exercise has to become an
essential part of your life—like eating, sleeping, and brushing your
teeth. No matter how busy you get, you must make the time to move
your body. This can be difficult sometimes, especially when your
regular schedule has been disrupted, but a sense of perspective and a
little long-range planning will make it happen. (For more about
taking fitness on the road, see Chapter 22.)

6   Don't push too hard. Many people find that a good way to stick to a
regular exercise program is to hold back just a little. Be sure you get
your required workout, but if you feel great after running three miles
and a wreck after running four, it may be a good idea to stay with
three—or maybe compromise at 3.5. Meeting a challenge gives you a
good feeling, but so does knowing you can do a bit more if necessary.
If you push yourself too hard, you may end up quitting altogether.

7   Keep records. Even if the last thing on earth you think you need is
more paperwork, keeping a daily exercise log can be instructive, even
inspirational. There's no set formula for the information you should
record; you might want to make a note of the date, what you did, and
how difficult it was, on a scale of 1 to 10. If you felt a twinge in your
knee, make a note of it; if you had some stomach trouble, write down
what you ate; you may begin to see an interesting pattern. You can
use the log to keep track of your weight as well.

8   Don't use exercise as punishment. There's nothing terribly wrong
with running an extra mile to burn off a piece of cake, but it's not a
healthy psychological pattern to develop. (Besides, a mile will take
care of only about a third of the cake!) You're much better exercising
regularly and consistently, rain or shine, cake or no cake.

9   Use the buddy system. Many people think that the best thing about exercise is the solitude, but there are plenty of others who really enjoy a little company. Some can't manage without a pal to spur them on or shame them into showing up. Fitness director Karma Kientzler combines fitness with friendship with a cycling buddy; one morning a week they spend an hour huffing and puffing and catching up on news together. Sharing a workout can present scheduling problems, but it can be a wonderful motivator. Sometimes you need a policeman more than a companion—someone to check up on you and make sure you're not slacking off.

10 Reward yourself. Fitness is its own reward, true, but there is nothing wrong with giving yourself a pat on the back—or something even nicer and more tangible, such as a new warm-up suit or a pedometer—for a job well done.

PUTTING IT IN WRITING

The idea of a "fitness contract" may seem a little silly, but the exercise physiologists here at the Ranch, who have co-signed many such contracts, think that they're remarkably effective in motivating people to succeed.

A contract can be helpful in several ways: it forces you to spell out your goals, clearly and specifically; it serves as a reminder of the commitment you made; and it makes you accountable for your behavior in a way you might not otherwise be. You can't just write it out and hide it in a drawer; you have to get someone to witness the document and keep a copy. Arrange to refer to the contract every month or so to monitor your progress. Your co-conspirator could be almost any objective third party: a friend, a doctor, a nutritionist, or an exercise instructor. Involving a spouse or a Significant Other may be a problem, though; we've seen instances in which a broken contract led to marital arguments.

Here's a sample of a contract created for one of our guests.

Fitness Contract

_____
(Date)

I,_____, hereby promise to:

1. Lose 46 pounds in one year.
2. Lose one pound per week.
3. Eat approximately 1500 calories per day.
4. Walk or bike a minimum of 30 continuous minutes at least four times a week.
5. Never go more than two days in a row without exercise.
6. Develop a plan to deal with stress in the office.
7. Do relaxation breathing exercises three times a day.

_____   _____
(Signature)   (Witness)

THE POINT SYSTEM

Another device we've had a lot of success with at the Ranch is the fitness point system. It's quite simple, and it's not unlike the food exchange system that many nutritionists use. Each fitness activity you're likely to choose is worth points, and you have to earn a certain number of points every month. Here's how the points break down:

ACTIVITY	UNIT	POINTS PER UNIT	POINTS PER HOUR
CYCLING	1 mile	1	14–22
	15 minutes	4	16
STATIONARY CYCLING	15 minutes	4	16
BRISK WALKING	1 mile	3	12–15
	15 minutes	3	12
HIKING	15 minutes	3	12
RUNNING	1 mile	3	15–30
SWIMMING	¼ mile	3	12–24
AEROBIC DANCE	15 minutes	3	12
SINGLES TENNIS	15 minutes	3–4	12–16
DOUBLES TENNIS	15 minutes	1–2	4–8
RACQUETBALL	15 minutes	3–4	12–16
CIRCUIT WEIGHTS	15 minutes	4	16
CROSS-COUNTRY SKIING	15 minutes	5	20
MINI TRAMPOLINE	15 minutes	3	12
ROWING MACHINE	15 minutes	4	16
WEIGHT LOSS	1 pound	5	—

THE PERSONAL TOUCH

Once upon a time only athletes and movie stars had personal trainers, but that's not so any more. These days plenty of regular folks opt for one-on-one exercise instruction. Personal trainers don't come cheap, however; an hour with a trainer will cost anything from $20 to $100-plus. For your money you get privacy, convenience, and a tailor-made fitness program. You also get discipline.

To find a trainer ask your doctor, your friends, your health club, and your local college or university. (You could be the term project for an eager phys ed or sportsmedicine major.) Ask for and check references before you make any kind of deal, and beware of rash promises. Spell out what you want from your workout. Most important of all, make sure that the chemistry is right between the two of you. If you don't feel comfortable with your trainer, find another one.

We help our guests work out the number of points they should be aiming for, but you should be able to do that for yourself. The minimum number of fitness points you should accumulate each month is 105, which you would just about earn if you walk for only a half-hour every other day.

We encourage people to give themselves behavioral points as well as activity points. For every day you achieve a certain specified goal—keep your food intake below 1500 calories, do your breathing exercises, drink eight glasses of water, eat breakfast, or meditate, to name a few you might pick—you get a point. It's best if you take on one behavior at a time. Work on breathing one month; breathing and drinking water the next; breathing, drinking water, and meditating the next; and so on.

We've found that a month is the ideal time frame in which to work. It's short enough to give you a reachable goal and long enough to give you some flexibility. Don't be surprised if you have a rush of activity toward the end of the month, when you have to play catch-up. Practically everyone using the point system does.

Here is a sample of a completed monthly point tally and a blank form so that you can calculate your own score. I. M. Fitt had 159 activity points and 22 behavioral points for the month. The dates that are circled are the ones on which Fitt did not eat after nine o'clock at night.

NAME I.M. FITT

MONTH AUGUST

YEAR 1988

Please fill in the **activities** and **points** EACH DAY.

DATE	ACTIVITY	DISTANCE/TIME	POINTS	CUMULATIVE POINTS
8-1	WALK	2 MILES / 40 MIN.	6	6
8-2	-	-	-	6
8-3	WALK	2 MILES / 40 MIN.	-	12
8-4	STA. CYCLE	30 MIN.	8	20
8-5	-	-	-	20
8-6	WALK	2 MILES / 39 MIN	6	26
8-7	-	-	-	26
8-8	SWIM/STA. CYCLE	1/4 MILE/14 MIN - 30MIN	3/8	37
8-9	-	-		37
8-10	WALK	2 MILES/40 MIN	6	43
8-11	WALK	2 MILES/40 MIN	6	49
8-12	TENNIS (DOUBLES)	60 MIN	8	57
8-13	-	-	-	57
8-14	SWIM	1/2 MILE · 32 MIN	6	63
8-15	STA. CYCLE	30 MIN	8	71
8-16	-	-	-	71
8-17	WALK	3 MILES/60 MIN.	9	80
8-18	WALK	2 MILES/37 MIN	6	86
8-19	STA. CYCLE	30 MIN.	8	94
8-20	-	-	-	94
8-21	TENNIS (DOUBLES)	60 MIN.	8	102
8-22	SWIM	1/2 MILE · 30 MIN.	6	108
8.23	WALK	2 MILES · 37 MIN	6	114
8.24	-	-	-	-
8.25	STA. CYCLE	45 MIN.	12	126
8.26	WALK	2 MILES/37 MIN	6	132
8.27	WALK	3 MILES/57 MIN	9	141

(153)	(21)	(180)
ACTIVITY PTS. +	NO. DAYS =	TOTAL POINTS

CANYON RANCH FITNESS PROGRAM

ACTIVITY LOG

NAME _____

MONTH _____

YEAR _____

Please fill in the **activities** and **points** EACH DAY.

DATE	ACTIVITY	DISTANCE/TIME	POINTS	CUMULATIVE POINTS

(_____)   (_____)   (_____)
ACTIVITY PTS.   +   NO. DAYS   =   TOTAL POINTS

7

How does aerobic exercise help you? Let us count the ways. It speeds up metabolism, enhances muscle endurance, and improves circulation and digestion. It does wonders for the heart, strengthening the heart muscle, enlarging the main heart chamber so that more blood is pumped per beat, and decreasing the resting heart rate. It keeps your weight down, gives you self-confidence, lets you sleep better, and relieves stress. Practically the only thing it doesn't do is windows.

Aerobic activity got its name, simply enough, because it uses air. The harder you breathe, the more oxygen you use (because it's necessary to pump the extra blood to the working muscles) and the more calories you burn. Most women use about 1.7 liters of oxygen a minute when they're working their hardest; men use about 3.4 liters. Using one liter of oxygen burns up five calories.

If you get short of air, such as when you sprint, for instance, you are exercising anaerobically, or without air. You can get a perfectly good workout from anaerobic exercise, but it takes longer. A vigorous game of squash, tennis, or racquetball (which are a combination of aerobic and anaerobic exercise), is a perfectly acceptable form of exercise, but aerobically speaking, 75 minutes of singles tennis and 60 minutes of squash and racquetball are equal to about 30 minutes of very brisk walking.

Your Target Heart Rate

The official definition of an aerobic exercise is one that raises your heart rate—the number of times it beats per minute—to within 60 to 85 percent of its capacity and keeps it there, at the

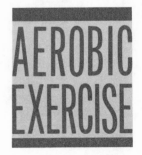

AEROBIC EXERCISE

"target heart rate," for a specified amount of time, usually 20 to 40 minutes. More specifically, the American College of Sportsmedicine says that if your target heart rate is 60 percent of maximum, you need 90 minutes of exercise for aerobic fitness; at 70 percent you need 40 minutes; and at 85 percent, 30 minutes will do.

When you embark on an aerobic exercise program, the first step is to calculate what your target heart rate is. One formula you may use, which takes into account your resting and maximum heart rates (Rest HR and Max HR), is known as Karvonen's Formula:

$$[(Max\ HR - Rest\ HR) \times (\%\ capacity)] + (Rest\ HR) = Target\ HR$$

If you don't know your maximum heart rate, an easy way to get a ballpark figure is with simple subtraction. The maximum heart rate for men is 205 minus half your age; the maximum heart rate for women is 220 minus your age.

To get a target heart rate range you simply multiply the maximum heart rate by 60 percent, 70 percent, and 85 percent. At the Ranch we post a target heart rate chart in all classes for easy reference. For obvious reasons, the numbers on it are estimates, but they can be useful as a guideline.

TARGET HEART RATES
(Ten Seconds)

AGE	60%		70%		85%	
	MEN	WOMEN	MEN	WOMEN	MEN	WOMEN
20–22	19	20	23	23	28	28
23–25	19	19	23	23	28	28
26–28	19	19	22	22	27	27
29–31	19	19	22	22	26	27
32–34	18	19	21	21	26	26
35–37	18	18	21	21	26	26
38–40	18	18	21	21	26	26
41–43	18	18	21	21	26	26
44–46	18	17	21	20	25	25
47–49	18	17	21	20	25	24
50–52	18	17	20	20	25	24
53–55	17	17	20	19	25	23
56–58	17	16	20	19	25	23
59–60	17	16	20	19	24	23
61–65	17	15	20	18	24	22
66–70	17	15	19	18	24	22
71–75	16	14	19	16	23	20

A normal resting heart rate is somewhere between 70 and 100 beats per minute, but some well-conditioned athletes have gotten theirs down as low as 50. In general, a relatively low resting heart rate is a sign of fitness—as you continue to exercise, your heart rate will probably go down—but that is not always the case. Some people, even unfit people, have unusually low resting heart rates. To complicate matters even more, your heart rate will vary from day to day and even hour to hour. When you're angry or excited or in pain, it may go up; depression or sleep brings it down. A true resting heart rate is measured as soon as you wake up in the morning before you get out of bed.

Measuring Your Heart Rate

All you need to calculate your heart rate is two fingers and a watch with a second hand. Press the index and middle fingers of one hand on the thumb side of the wrist of the other, palm side up, find your pulse, and count the number of beats you feel in a ten-second period. Multiply that number by six and you'll have the number of beats per minute. If the pulse in your wrist is not strong enough to measure, try your carotid artery. Press your two fingertips lightly but firmly on the side of your neck just under the jawbone and count the beats.

If aerobic exercise is a new adventure for you, you would do well to monitor your heart rate for a while, until you get to know what it feels like to be in your target heart rate range. Eventually you'll be able to forget about watches and mathematics and carotid arteries and listen to your body. If your breathing seems right (rapid but not labored) and you're sweating enough, you'll know you're getting a good workout.

Burning Calories

The most effective fat-burning exercise is aerobic, for the simple reason that calorie expenditure is, as we explained earlier, determined by the amount of oxygen we use during exercise; one liter of oxygen burned uses five calories. In the ideal aerobic exercise workout you'll burn up at least 300 calories. To give you an idea of what that means the following chart, prepared by the National Institutes of Health, lists the number of calories that are burned by a 150-pound person during various forms of exercise. Someone weighing 100 pounds will burn one third fewer calories; a 200-pounder will burn a third more.

ACTIVITY	CALORIES BURNED PER HOUR
BICYCLING, 6 MPH	240
BICYCLING, 12 MPH	410
CROSS-COUNTRY SKIING	700
JOGGING, 5.5 MPH	740
JOGGING, 7 MPH	920
JUMPING ROPE	750
RUNNING IN PLACE	650
RUNNING, 10 MPH	1280
SWIMMING, 25 YDS/MIN	275
SWIMMING, 50 YDS/MIN	500
TENNIS, SINGLES	400
WALKING, 2 MPH	240
WALKING, 3 MPH	320
WALKING, 4.5 MPH	440

THE BEST AEROBIC EXERCISE

All aerobic exercises—whether they're on that chart or not—are good for you if you do them vigorously enough to give your heart a good workout. The best exercise is the one that you are the most likely to do consistently. Jogging is wonderful, but if you hate to do it, you'll eventually stop. A stationary bike can be the perfect home exercise tool, but if cycling bores you to tears, the bike will soon become something to drape your shirts on. Find something you like that's convenient to do and do it regularly. Better yet, find two aerobic activities you enjoy and switch off from time to time.

At the Ranch we like them all: walking, running, hiking, bicycling, swimming, jumping rope, aerobic dance, and every manner of exercise that involves equipment. Perhaps the following descriptions will help you make your choice.

WALKING

At Canyon Ranch the day begins at seven o'clock, when virtually all the guests assemble at the tennis courts to warm up for the brisk morning walk. Like all the activities at the Ranch, the walk is optional, but most people say that they wouldn't dream of missing it, even when the four-miler is hilly and the leader seems determined to set a new speed record. Beginners usually try the one- or two-mile walks, and there's a three-miler as well. Whatever the mileage of the walk, everyone gets some kind of aerobic workout to start the day.

Walking is one of the best all-around fitness activities. It burns calories; if you walk only 15 miles a week—three miles a day, five days a week—you'll burn anywhere from 1000 to 1500 calories, depending on how much you weigh and how fast you walk. It strengthens the back and is especially good for the legs, hips, and lower abdomen. If you pump your arms when you walk, it can also work the arms, shoulders, sides, back, and chest. Like all weight-bearing exercises, walking makes the bones stronger and more dense. (That's why weight-bearing exercise may help to prevent osteoporosis.) Unlike running and the other more ballistic exercises, walking doesn't cause trauma to the bones and joints; walkers are not likely to suffer from stress fractures or tendinitis, injuries that are quite common among runners. If you're recovering from an injury, if you have arthritis, or if you're very out of shape, walking may be one of the few exercises you *can* do.

Studies show that a regular walking program lowers your blood pressure and resting heart rate, decreases blood fats, and increases HDL cholesterol, the kind that clears fatty deposits out of your arteries. And there's nothing to it: all you have to remember is heel-toe, keep your arms moving rhythmically, and don't bump into anything.

SPEED

The only problem with walking as a fitness activity is that you have to be sure to do it fast enough. (One of the least pleasant surprises that many of our guests receive is finding out that they've been walking much too slowly at home.) Beginning walkers will not have a problem reaching their target heart rate, but as you get in better shape, reaching 75 percent of your maximum heart rate and keeping it there for a minimum of 20 minutes will become more of a challenge. To increase the demands on your body you'll have to walk faster, drive your arms more vigorously, walk uphill, or do all three.

Fitness walking is generally considered to be somewhere between 3.5 and 5 miles per hour, but most people have no idea how fast they walk. The following chart, prepared by the Berkeley Wellness Letter, can help you calculate your speed. Before you can use it, though, you have to count the number of steps you take per minute. (Note: this chart is based on a 2.5-foot stride. If yours is closer to 3 feet, you don't need the chart. Just divide the number of strides per minute by 30 to get your miles per hour.)

STEPS PER MINUTE	MPH
70	2.0
90	2.5
105	3.0
120	3.5
140	4.0
160	4.5
175	5.0
190	5.5

WALKING UPHILL

When you're walking along briskly, engaged in animated conversation with a companion, and all of a sudden you're out of breath, it's probably not because you're getting tired. It's more likely that you've started walking uphill. *Prevention* magazine says that when you walk four mph for a half hour on level ground, you burn about 220 calories; if you walk up a 5 percent grade (for every 100 feet you travel the ground rises five), it's more than 300 calories; a 10 percent grade makes it 425 calories; and a 20 percent incline burns more than 600. It's no wonder you get out of breath climbing stairs; that's a whopping 50 percent grade.

Some walkers take the uphill route because it's the most efficient use of time; instead of walking for an hour on level ground, they can walk uphill for 30 minutes. There may be a price to pay for those extra burned calories or saved minutes, however. Walking uphill is a little harder on the legs and buttocks, and it's much more demanding on the lungs. To keep from hurting yourself start with a gradual slope and work up slowly and steadily.

FOOTWEAR

A good walking shoe has a firm heel counter, a wide or flared heel base, a high, wide toe box, and lots of cushioning. They're supportive but light, flexible but firm, and made of natural fibers. Since you may not even know what a heel counter or a toe box *is,* you're probably going to need some advice. The good news is that you won't have to go very far; everywhere you look, walking shoes are in.

When you are picking out a pair of walking shoes, don't make the commonest mistake: buying shoes that are too small. Make allowances for the thick socks you'll be wearing and the fact that your feet swell— sometimes as much as a full size—when you've been walking for a while. Keep in mind that you need to be able to flex your foot. If you have flat feet, high arches or especially narrow or wide feet or if you overpronate when you walk (your ankles turn in), select a pair of shoes that compensates for those imperfections.

WHAT ABOUT WEIGHTS?

Hand and ankle weights are a mixed blessing. On the one hand they provide additional cardiovascular and muscular benefits to the walker; on the other, because they throw you a little off balance, they make you more susceptible to injuries. All things considered, you're probably better off without the weights, especially when you realize that in order to burn a significant number of extra calories, you would have to carry weights equal to 20 percent of your body weight. Most 130-pound women would find 13 extra pounds per ankle something of an impediment.

HIKING

"Would you visit London and not see Buckingham Palace? Would you go to Paris and not see the Eiffel Tower? Would you come to Tucson and not visit the mountains?"

That's how Phyllis Hochman began her letter to Mel Zuckerman back in 1979. Her purpose in writing was to persuade Mel to start a hiking program at Canyon Ranch. Phyllis is wildly enthusiastic about the benefits and joys of hiking, and for good reason. Hiking practically saved her life.

Diagnosed as having severe scoliosis at the age of 13, Phyllis had been inactive all her life. At 35 she was told that there was a 50-50 chance that she would be wheelchair-bound by the time she was 50. At 40 she was going downhill fast. Then, in her mid-forties, for reasons she can't quite explain, Phyllis decided that instead of becoming an invalid she was going to make herself strong. She gave up chilly New York winters for the warm Arizona sun and got physical.

The next thing she knew, she was a card-carrying member of the senior citizens' faction of the Southern Arizona Hiking Club, who hiked four or five miles every week. For a long time she brought up the rear, came home totally wiped out, and took to her bed for 24 hours, but eventually she got stronger. With each passing month she was able to climb faster and recuperate more quickly. Needless to say, on her fiftieth birthday Phyllis did not need a wheelchair; if anything, she needed a new pair of hiking shoes.

It didn't take much to persuade Mel Zuckerman that hiking belonged on the Canyon Ranch fitness program (he had spent some of his happiest times hiking in the mountains himself), and since the day Phyllis's letter arrived, more than 18,000 people have hiked about 80,000 miles with her or her staff. Every day a few vans full of guests venture "off-campus" to explore the nearby mountains—and get a great workout.

THE BENEFITS

Think of hiking as uphill walking with scenery. It's aerobically demanding, more so than just about any other exercise, but it's also *real;* climbing a real hill offers challenges and satisfactions that running around a track or pedaling a stationary bike simply can't give you. Another great thing about hiking is that it accommodates all fitness levels. Not everyone can rush up the side of a steep mountain without breathing hard, but everyone can hike somewhere at some speed. If you pace yourself properly and know your limitations, hiking is something you can take with you into your old age.

HOW TO DO IT

Always start a hike slowly, letting your blood start to circulate and your muscles get warm. Once you establish your pace, keep it steady. For maximum aerobic benefits, keep moving, however slowly. When you walk uphill, make sure your heel hits the ground first. Walking on your toes will give you tight, sore muscles the next day. On the way downhill, keep your knees flexed and soft. Cool down by strolling the last half mile of a hike.

Dress in loose, unrestrictive layers of clothing—you'll be a lot warmer on the way up that hill than you will be on the way down—and protect your head from the elements with a hat.

Even more important than protecting your head is, of course, protecting your feet. Wear two pairs of socks—first a thinner one, made of nylon or some other synthetic fiber (look for "wicking action," fabric that wicks the sweat away from the foot), then a thicker pair, made of wool—to help reduce friction between your feet and shoes or boots. (Coating your feet with petroleum jelly will also cut down on friction.) A good running shoe will do perfectly well for hiking, provided it has plenty of support, adequate cushioning, and a lot of room in the toe. If you become serious about hiking, you'll probably want to graduate to hiking shoes or boots.

RUNNING

A lot of people who help run Canyon Ranch—chief operating officer Bill Day and president Jerry Cohen, for instance—do their serious exercising somewhere else. When they want a workout, they're not likely to be found in the gyms or the aerobics classes or even on the hiking trails. Like hundreds of thousands of other people in the country, they're out running.

Perhaps the most enthusiastic runner in the bunch is exercise physiologist Eric Chesky, who waxes poetic about running and gets downright cranky when people say bad things about it. He acknowledges that not everyone has the physique, or the stamina, to run a marathon, but he sees no reason why anyone who wants to take up running can't do it for 30 minutes at a time four times a week.

Anything walking can do, running can do better, or at least faster; it burns calories, exercises the legs and buttocks, and gives the heart and lungs a thorough workout. It also relieves stress and clears the head; many people say that they are at their most creative when they're running.

HOW TO DO IT

Running is not without its hazards, however, as Eric would be the first to admit. It's a high-impact sport, after all, and that means that creaky bones and joints can take something of a beating if you don't do it right. Here are some of Eric's pointers:

♦ Land on your heel and push off with your toes, propelling yourself forward. The faster you go, the more time you'll spend on your toes.

♦ Your motion should be forward, not up and down or side to side. Put one foot directly in front of the other in the center of your body. You can cut down on the impact by reducing vertical displacement.

♦ After pushing off with your toes, bring your knees forward. Keep your feet low to the ground and throw your heel out so that it drops right under your knee. Your angle of hip flexion should be only 8 to 10 degrees. Don't overstride.

♦ Relax your upper body and lean forward slightly.

♦ Keep a 90-degree bend in your arm and your hands loosely cupped—as if you were holding a piece of paper between your index finger and thumb. Drive your arms firmly but not too energetically. The more vigorous your arm motion is, the faster you run.

♦ Run on the softest, most level surface you can find. Dirt and grass are particularly kind to the joints. Running on sand or on too steep a slope can be hazardous to your health.

THE JOG-WALK PROGRAM

WEEK	FREQUENCY (TIMES PER WEEK)	DURATION (MINUTES) WALK X JOG	TOTAL TIME
1	3–5	5 × 1	20
2	3–5	5 × 1	25
3	3–5	4 × 2	25
4	3–5	4 × 2	30
5	3–5	3 × 3	30
6	3–5	3 × 4	30
7	3–5	3 × 4	35
8	3–5	2 × 4	35
9	3–5	2 × 4	40
10	3–5	1 × 5	40

You're never too old or too unfit to try running if you want to, but everyone must take it slowly at first; if you're not used to running, you probably won't be able to keep it up for more than a few minutes at first. Everyone progresses at a different pace, of course, but the Jog-Walk Program, outlined here, can be useful for almost any beginner. Use it as a guide but don't be bound by it. If you think you're ready to move on to the next step before the program suggests, go to it.

CYCLING

"Today's runner is tomorrow's cyclist."

That's what Frank Lister says, and he should know. He's the man who runs the Canyon Ranch biking program.

The Bicycle Federation of America says that there are more than 40 million adult cyclists. A lot of people who rode bikes as kids are rediscovering the sport, and many of them have indeed turned to cycling after being injured on the running track. People have taken up the sport to burn calories, build endurance, reduce stress, and get out in the fresh air for a good time. Biking is good for the quadriceps, the abdominal muscles, the heart, and the lungs. Frank Lister says it's good for the soul too. He calls it "cycle therapy."

There is nothing wrong with stationary cycling (see page 93), but for Frank Lister, and an increasing number of the Canyon Ranch guests, there is nothing quite like bicycling in the great outdoors. What makes that kind of derring-do possible in this part of the world is the mountain bike, the weird-looking bike with the fat tires, soft saddles, and wide handlebars. Sometimes referred to as the Jeep of bicycles, the mountain bike is stable, comfortable, and easy to ride. Its strong frame and 15 gears allow you to get to places you never thought you could reach. (However, you can't get there quite so quickly as you might on a regular bike, since your upright position makes you less aerodynamically efficient.) Designed for uphill work and especially resistant to sand and gravel, the fat-tired bikes can go anywhere, but many city folks prefer a scaled-down version: the city bike. This variation has 10 instead of 15 gears and a slightly narrower tire, but otherwise it has the same features and advantages as the mountain bike.

HOW TO DO IT

Regardless of what kind of bike you use, to get an aerobic workout you need to pedal about five miles in 20 minutes. The Bicycle Federation of America recommends that you not increase your mileage more than 20 percent a week.

Here are some of Frank Lister's tips on proper cycling form:

♦ Stay loose. Inexperienced riders tend to grip the handlebars too hard, which makes for tight shoulder and back muscles, and hunch over too far, which causes low back pain. Relax your arms and shoulders and move around on the saddle every once in a while. When you feel yourself tightening up, get off the bike for a minute and stretch your back, shoulders, hamstrings, and quadriceps. (See Chapter 8 for stretching exercises.)

♦ Arrange your seat correctly. Cycling can be rough on the knees, especially if your seat is not at the right height. Adjust your seat so that your leg is almost fully extended at the bottom of the pedal stroke, with the ball of your foot on the pedal.

♦ Don't ride in too high a gear. This is a mistake many cyclists make, thinking that the harder they make the workout, the more beneficial it will be. Not true. It's better for your heart (and your knees) if you stay in a lower gear, somewhere between 60 and 100 revolutions per minute. Keep your cadence even.

♦ Don't forget your upper body. Cycling is great for the quads, but it doesn't do much to strengthen the upper body. Upper body strength is important for overall fitness, and it can make cycling much easier, too. Supplement your cycling regimen with calisthenics, push-ups, pull-ups, or working with light weights.

♦ Stay out of heavy traffic. Exercise is supposed to relieve stress, not create it.

WHAT TO WEAR

Cyclists like the layered look: cycling tights with sweat pants over them; a T-shirt covered by a sweatshirt covered by a windbreaker. On cool days you'll need warm wool gloves and something that covers your ears. The most important accessory, if not always the most fetching, is a helmet.

The best thing for your feet are bicycle touring shoes, which have a steel plate from about the ball of the foot to the heel. The foot is supported, but the ball remains flexible. Cleated shoes are all right too, but you can't walk around in them as you can in touring shoes. Toe clips are optional, but they're great if you want to go as fast as possible; Frank says that the clips increase your efficiency by about 30 percent.

JUMPING ROPE

For some people jumping rope is one of several fitness activities, since it can be done in all seasons, all weather, and even in small hotel rooms.

If it's too cold to run and the swimming pool is closed, you can always break out the jump rope. Jumping rope gives you aerobic strength and muscular endurance, and it improves your balance, agility, and coordination. As if that wasn't enough, it can also give you something of a cognitive workout as well, as you force yourself to concentrate on your steps. If you don't believe that, try taking the Canyon Ranch Jump Rope class without paying attention.

HOW TO DO IT

Jumping rope raises the heart rate very quickly, so unless you are quite aerobically fit already, you should start a jump rope program very slowly. Don't worry at first about getting in your 20-minute aerobic workout, although that should be your aim. Jump for a minute, walk in place for a minute, then jump for a minute. Build up to jumping for two minutes and walking for one, then jumping for three and walking for one, and so on. It may take a few weeks or even a few months to build up to 20 straight minutes.

Here are a few other things to keep in mind:

♦ The best surface for jumping rope is a wood floor. Try to find a vacant basketball or racquetball court.

♦ Take it slow. It's harder to jump slowly than it is to jump fast. The slower you jump, the more power and strength you need.

♦ Don't look at your feet. Stand erect and jump when you hear the rope hit the ground.

♦ Land on the balls of your feet, not your heels.

THE ROPE

One of the best things about jumping rope is that the top-of-the-line equipment costs only about 20 dollars. When you're shopping for a rope, make sure that the handles reach your armpits when you stand on the middle of the rope. (If you're 6 feet tall, a 9½-foot rope is about right; an 8-footer is better for shorter people.) The rope should be heavy enough to develop a good rhythm; clothesline rope is so light it tends to float. The jump rope instructors at the Ranch swear by the Lifeline jump rope, which has plastic links and replaceable handles.

WHAT TO WEAR

Anything that gives you freedom of movement, especially under the arms, is fine for jumping rope. Leotards, shorts, and sweats work particularly well, and a headband usually comes in handy. The best shoes for the job are basketball shoes, especially high tops, since they are designed for quick starts and stops, 180 degree turns, and pivoting on a wood floor.

If you do your jumping on something harder than wood, such as concrete, you may need padded socks and shock absorbers in your shoes.

SWIMMING

There is only one exercise that refreshes you and cools you down at the same time it heats up your heart rate and works nearly every muscle in your body. It's the same exercise that burns calories, improves your posture and muscular endurance, develops long, lean, flexible muscles, and usually requires a silly-looking cap. It's also fitness director Karma Kientzler's favorite sport.

Exercising in the water has many good points, but perhaps the best is that unlike some of the other forms of aerobic exercise, it can be done and enjoyed by everyone. Because water absorbs up to 80 percent of a person's body weight, it's great for people who are overweight or pregnant. Because the buoyancy of the water prevents any forceful impact on your bones and joints, it's highly recommended for disabled people and others who do not have the full range of movement. (Some arthritis sufferers have experienced virtual miracles in the water.) Water allows the muscles to stretch, giving you a greater range of motion without the risk of sprains or tears. You can do things in the water that you could never do on land. Exercising in the water also has a therapeutic effect. Almost everyone feels relaxed as well as invigorated after a water workout.

If it weren't for ear infections, green hair, and the fact that most of us don't have the space or the money for our own pools, swimming would be just about perfect.

HOW TO DO IT

A good swimming program calls for about 30 minutes of continuous swimming four times a week, but it will take you some time to build up to that. At the beginning, swim a few laps, rest, swim a few more, and rest again. Shorten your rest periods until you can swim a half-hour without stopping. Any pool will do for a workout, but of course, larger pools are best because you don't have to turn around so often.

The best all-around stroke for achieving a good cardiovascular and muscular workout is the forward crawl, or freestyle swimming. The side stroke and breast stroke aren't as vigorous, but either can be used as a change of pace. A complete workout will include the backstroke, breast stroke, butterfly stroke, side stroke, and the crawl. When you're doing pool aerobics, aim for a full range of motion. Instead of doing many fast, short moves, it's more effective for your heart and your muscles if you make the motions broad and slow.

Be sure to warm up before and cool down after your swimming workout, with stretching exercises and slow, relaxed swimming. Don't forget that even with all that water around you can get dehydrated when you swim, so you'll need to replenish your missing fluids after you're finished.

A SWIMMER'S HEART RATE

Your heart beats more slowly when you're in the water—about 15 beats per minute slower than when you're on land—because the swimming position enables your heart to pump blood more easily. This means that in order to get the aerobic benefits you're looking for from an aerobic workout, you don't have to strive for such a high target heart rate. In fact, if you reach the same target heart rate in the water as you do when you work out on dry land, you are probably working too hard. To find your maximum heart rate for swimming men should subtract half their age from 195, and women should subtract their age from 205; then both should work to within 60 to 85 percent of that new number.

FLUGELS

The aquatics program at the Ranch is big and getting bigger all the time. The Aqua Trim and Pool Aerobics classes are extremely popular, especially in our Arizona summers, and the new Lap Swimming and Stroke Technique classes are gaining fast. The class that is making the biggest splash, however, is Flugels.

In Flugels class you can't sink, and it's difficult to swim, because attached to your hands and ankles are Flugels—the German word for wings—specially designed flotation devices that use the buoyancy and resistance of the water to increase the intensity of an exercise. Flugels have proved to be highly effective in building muscular endurance, enhancing flexibility, improving cardiovascular efficiency, and developing better balance and coordination. They're also a great equalizer: everyone, young or old, in and out of shape, feels like a fish out of water when he puts them on for the first time.

THE HAZARDS

There's no way to get around the fact that pools contain chlorine, and chlorine is murder on the hair and the eyes. To protect your hair spread a couple of drops of mineral oil or baby oil in the palm of your hands and coat your hair with it before you get in the pool; wear a bathing cap, preferably a silicone cap; and shampoo right after you get out of the pool.

If your hair becomes discolored, try one of the many anti-chlorine shampoos, such as Aloe-Rid, which is especially effective.

A pair of tight-fitting goggles will probably protect your eyes. If they sting even with the goggles, talk to the club manager; the PH balance of the pool may be out of whack. If your eyes are red and sore from swimming, try some of the "artificial tears" products available in your drugstore or try an herbal remedy. See page 59 for herbal eye care remedies.

Low-Impact Aerobics

For the last ten years or so Americans have had a love affair with aerobics, and we have the injuries to prove it: shin splints, bad knees, sore hips, and chronic lower back problems, not to mention torn ligaments, tendinitis, and more than a few sprained ankles. As we often do when we find something that we like, we overdid it.

As we now know, ballistic movements—especially the indiscriminate flinging of the arms and deep knee bends—put stress on the joints, and they may cause small tears in the muscles. Jumping up and down can create problems too, for obvious reasons; you land with a force equal to about three times your weight.

So low-impact aerobics (also called "soft" or "nonballistic" aerobics) was born. In low-impact aerobics your body stays closer to the floor than in conventional aerobics, with the body's pressure against the floor used to create resistance and condition muscles. So instead of jumping jacks, hopping, running in place, and high leg kicks, you get sliding, lunging, marching, leg swings, leg lifts, side-stepping, and dance combinations. In general low-impact relies on fast footwork or wide, strong movements for the legs and torso combined with lots of arm work. One foot remains on the floor at all times.

The goal of low-impact aerobics is to get your heart pumping with a minimum of strain on the joints. This calls for exaggerated movements of the larger muscle groups; you keep one foot on the floor, but you lift the other one high, then add arm motions to get your heart pumping even harder. The lower you bend to the floor and the higher you hold your arms over your head, the greater the workout. By keeping your arms in constant motion you can increase your cardiovascular workout by as much as 20 percent without straining your legs or feet.

Some fitness fanatics resist the concept of low-impact aerobics because it sounds wimpy, but that could not be further from the truth. As our fitness instructors warn our guests before class, low impact does *not* mean low energy.

FINDING A CLASS

When aerobics classes are bad, they're horrid. At best they can be a waste of your time; at worst they can result in injuries. Here are a few tips on finding a good one:

♦ Check the floor. No matter how careful you are about low-impact, the wrong kind of floor can be the ruin of your joints. The worst ones are carpet-covered cement. The best are hardwood, ideally with an air space or a sponge layer beneath.

♦ Look for a well-balanced workout. All classes should include a warm-up period, an aerobic workout, and a cool-down period. A 45-minute session should break down to roughly 15 minutes of warm-up and stretching, 20 minutes in which your heart rate is up to its optimal range, and 10 minutes of cooling off. The exercises should be varied and should cover all muscles, large and small.

♦ Give it time. Aerobic dance classes burn calories and give you energy, but they can also make you feel like a real klutz. More than a few people have walked out of a class more frustrated than fit, because they couldn't keep up with the complicated steps. There is more to an aerobics dance class than a cardiovascular workout; if it's done right, it stimulates the brain too. Don't stay with a class that's impossibly hard but don't give up too easily either. Sometimes it takes two or three classes with the same instructor to get the hang of things.

FOOTWEAR

In our aerobics classes we ask our guests to wear shoes for support and stability. Running shoes have too much tread to allow for movement in all directions (and they're designed to accept impact only on the heel), but tennis-type shoes and special aerobics shoes are fine.

AEROBIC EXERCISE EQUIPMENT

One of the busiest places at Canyon Ranch is Gym 2. That's where we keep the aerobic exercise equipment. Day and night people are in the gym, pedaling, rowing, cross country skiing, and running in place. Like everyone else, our guests love machines, in gyms, in health clubs, and in their own homes.

It is estimated that in 1986 Americans bought more than a billion dollars worth of home exercise equipment. The appeal of a home gym is obvious: the hours are reasonable, you don't have to wait in line for a machine, the weather is always pleasant, and you don't end up with rocks in your shoes. If you feel like it, you can even work out in your pajamas.

However, when it comes to shopping, it can be a jungle out there.

If you decide to stock your home gym with some major pieces of exercise equipment, such as a treadmill, exercise bike, rowing machine, mini trampoline, or cross-country ski machine, shop around before you buy. Catalog shopping is fine but only if you've tried out the exact model yourself. Beware of very cheap merchandise, although you may find some real bargains in the classifieds of your newspaper. Slightly used machines and discounted floor models can be terrific. Be sure you know exactly how to use whatever it is you decide to buy.

In the final analysis, all types of aerobic exercise equipment are good, provided you use the equipment properly and it allows you to get your heart rate into the target zone and keep it there for 30 minutes. After that, it's just a matter of taste. If you like more than one machine but don't have the space or cash to buy both, find a neighbor to share with; you buy one, he'll buy the other, and you can arrange visitation rights.

TREADMILLS

Being able to take fitness walks or go jogging regardless of the weather or the time of day gives you a wonderful feeling of freedom. Treadmills give you that and more. They can take you up and down hills, speed you up and slow you down, even follow a pre-programmed regimen. Inclined treadmills are wonderful aerobic workout providers, and they help you keep your calves, hamstrings, quadriceps, and buttocks in shape. All this comes at a price, of course: A good treadmill, with adjustable speed and elevation, will cost around $3000.

MINI TRAMPOLINES

Rebounding on a mini trampoline is an imperfect exercise—the trampoline does a little too much of the work to make it perfect—but it can be good as a supplementary fitness activity, and besides, it's fun. Look for a sturdy frame and legs, a tough surface, and heavy-duty springs. Square or rectangular trampolines are generally more stable than round ones. They cost anywhere from $25 to $100.

STATIONARY BICYCLES

It's not difficult to understand why stationary bikes are so popular. They're aerobically demanding, easy on the joints, and good for the thighs, hamstrings, hips, and buttocks. All that and you can read a magazine or watch the news while you work out.

Look for a heavy flywheel for smooth pedaling, a comfortable seat, foot straps or toe clips, an adjustable workload, and measurement devices for speed, distance, or (best of all) RPMs. Ergometers, which calculate how hard you're working in watts or calories, are necessary only if you want to know those things. A good basic bike will cost $250 to $500. An ergometer-equipped model will run you $500 to $1000.

ROWING MACHINES

Pound for pound, this machine uses more muscle groups and burns more calories than any other piece of exercise equipment except the cross-country ski machine. If you use it correctly, it gives you an excellent aerobic workout and strengthens both the upper and the lower body.

Many people complain that rowing machines hurt their backs, but that's probably because they're using the machines incorrectly. To begin the exercise sit in an upright position. When you move forward, keep your back straight and stretch your shoulders only slightly. As you pull back, use only your legs, shoulders, and arms. Your back should remain straight, relaxed, and uninvolved in the rowing motion. At the end of the pull, come to an upright position again; don't lean all the way back.

If you decide to get a rowing machine of your own, look for one that sits solidly on the floor and has smooth-moving oars. The seat should be comfortable, and it too should move easily on wheels or ball bearings. The foot rests should pivot. A good basic model costs $250 to $400-plus.

CROSS-COUNTRY SKI MACHINES

If you want a good laugh, watch someone who is trying one of these machines for the first time. It definitely takes practice to master a cross-country ski machine, but it's well worth the time and effort. These machines, which use every major muscle group without straining any of them, give you a great aerobic workout, and they're excellent for improving stamina. Models that use cords for hand movements seem to provide a more strenuous workout than those with poles. A good one costs about $600.

t's easy to see why stretching is the most overlooked component of fitness. First of all, it's too easy; you can stretch for an hour and never even break a sweat. Second, you can't really see the results—no thinner thighs or pumped-up pecs. There is no question about it: stretching is a distinctively un-flashy form of exercise. Stretching keeps you flexible, and there's nothing particularly glamorous about being flexible.

Flexibility, the body's ability to use muscles and joints through their full range of movement, is not in itself a sign of fitness. You can be fit and not be flexible, just as you can be flexible without being fit. Flexibility falls into the category of prevention, since it prepares the muscles for movement or activity and repairs some of the damage done by strenuous exercise. Exercise contracts the muscles; stretching is designed to lengthen them. When you stretch a muscle (or, more specifically, the connective tissue between the muscles), you feel resistance, like the tension of a stretched rubber band. Eventually, over time, that tension diminishes, and the muscle lengthens.

A regular program of gentle stretching can make a world of difference in the way you feel. Stretching relaxes the mind and tunes up the body; it can reduce muscle tension, promote circulation, prevent injuries, and make you more coordinated. What's more, it feels great. If you exercise regularly, stretching will prevent injuries and let you work up to your form, but even if you don't run or play tennis or do aerobics on a regular basis, you should make stretching a part of your life.

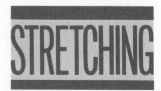

How Flexible Are You?

Raise your right arm and reach down your back as far as you can. At the same time place your left arm behind your back and try to touch the fingers of your right hand. (If this doesn't work, try it on the other side.) If your fingers touch, your arms and shoulders are fairly flexible.

Now lie on your back on a firm surface (a bench or a sturdy coffee table will do) with your knees bent over the edge and your feet on the floor. Keeping one leg in place, pull the other knee into your chest and hold it with both hands. Try it with the other leg. If you can't keep your lowered leg in place easily or if you feel discomfort in the groin area, you aren't very loose in the hips.

Now try to touch your toes without bending your knees. If you can do it easily and your lower back rounds when you bend over, you're fairly flexible. If you can't quite manage it and your back flattens out when you try, you're tight.

These exercises probably didn't tell you anything you didn't already know. Anyone who has ever tried to crawl into the back seat of a two-door car has a pretty good idea of how flexible he is. Some people are born loose; others are born tight. In general, women are more flexible than men, and young people more limber than old, but after that all bets are off. Many otherwise fit people are stiff as boards, and there are plenty of out-of-shape folks who can assume the lotus position.

Still, everyone can increase flexibility through stretching, and if you want to monitor your progress, it's a good idea to know where you started. The best way to do that is with the Sit and Reach Test, which measures the flexibility of the hamstrings and the muscles in the lower back.

THE SIT AND REACH TEST

You'll need a ruler, a box or step 8 to 12 inches high, and a friend. Tape the ruler to the top of the box so that it extends six inches in front of it. After warming up (run in place and pump your arms for a minute or two) sit with the soles of your bare feet flat against the box. Without bending your knees reach as far forward toward the box as you can without straining. Ask your friend to tell you how far along the ruler you were able to reach. Your flexibility rating is as follows:

UNDER 4	Poor
4 TO 9	Fair
9 TO 12	Good
OVER 12	Excellent

How to Stretch

There are three basic ways to stretch a muscle. The first is *ballistic,* in which you stretch to the limit and perform quick, repetitive bouncing movements. This kind may actually shorten your muscles and increase the chance of soreness or injury. The second is *contract-relax* stretching, in which you contract a muscle against a resistance, then relax into a static extension of the muscle. This kind is quite effective for increasing a muscle's flexibility, but it can be complicated to master, and it often calls for a partner. And then there's *static* stretching, in which you gradually extend a muscle through its full range of movement until you feel some resistance or the beginning of discomfort; hold the maximum position for 3 to 30 seconds; relax the muscle; and repeat it several times. The kind of stretching we recommend at Canyon Ranch is static.

As you practice your stretches, keep in mind that form is all. How you stretch is much more important than how much you stretch. Always relax into a stretch, then gradually increase the tension by stretching a little more. Breathe slowly and deeply. Never hold your breath or stretch to the point at which you can't breathe normally. And don't bounce; your motion should be gradual and relaxed. A stretch should be held for at least three seconds.

Remember that everyone's ability to stretch is very different, so don't let your competitive spirit get in the way of your good sense. Proper stretching means stretching within your own limits. Too much or too vigorous stretching can do more harm than good. Stretching is supposed

WHEN TO STRETCH

Before, during, or after exercise? The debate goes on and on. The best time to stretch a muscle is when it is warm and mobile, but that doesn't mean that you have to go through a whole workout before you limber up. Warm up quickly by running in place or riding a stationary bike for a couple of minutes. This movement increases your blood flow and raises muscle temperature, both of which are vital for muscle elasticity. When a muscle is cold, stretching it may cause a strain. After you've worked out, concentrate on stretching the muscle groups you just used to keep them from stiffening up.

to feel good. If you feel pain, stop. And don't give up. Even the stiffest, creakiest, least limber person in the world can eventually loosen up. Most people see results in a matter of a few weeks.

STRETCHES, HEAD TO TOE

A well-rounded exercise regimen will include a stretching session three or four times a week for something between 10 and 20 minutes. A stretching program should stretch specific muscles used in your sport or fitness activity as well as the general muscle groups: if you've been cycling, spend extra time on your quadriceps; if you're a runner, stretch your hamstrings; tennis players should concentrate on the upper back, shoulders, neck, and calves. Isolate the muscles you want to stretch. The more concentrated your efforts are, the more effective the stretch will be.

NECK STRETCHES
◆ Tilt your head as if you're trying to touch your ear to your shoulder. Exhale and hold the stretch for a few seconds. Inhale and try it on the other side. Do each side six to eight times.
◆ Turn your head from side to side, as if you're looking over your shoulder. Inhale as you turn and hold the position for a few seconds when you've turned as far as you can go. Do this six to eight times on each side.

SHOULDER AND UPPER BACK STRETCHES
◆ Pull your shoulders back, up, forward, and down six to eight times. Then reverse directions, going forward, up, back, and down. Inhale as you go up; exhale as you go down.
◆ Shrug your shoulders up as high as they can go, then slowly pull them down as far as you can. Repeat five times. Inhale as your shoulders go up; exhale as they go down.
◆ Grab your left shoulder with your right hand and cradle your right elbow in your left hand. Release your shoulder, relax your right arm, and pull your right arm toward the left and onto your chest. Hold the stretch for 20 or 30 seconds. Reverse arms. Repeat three times.
◆ Clasp your hands together behind you, lacing your fingers together. Pull your hands toward the ground and squeeze your elbows toward each other. Hold the stretch for 20 or 30 seconds.

CHEST/SHOULDER STRETCH
◆ With your arms at your sides stand with your back to a waist-high chair or bar. Reach behind you, grasping the surface of the bar with your

palms down and your thumbs pointing away from your body. Keeping your elbows straight, slowly drop to a kneeling position until you feel the stretch in your shoulders and upper chest. If this hurts, move your hands farther apart and try it again.

WAIST STRETCHES

♦ Face forward and, without bending your knees, slide your left hand down the outside of your left leg as far as you can without feeling any pain. Hold the stretch for 20 to 30 seconds and then slowly bring your arm back up. (To increase the stretch raise your right arm over your head.) Now slide your right hand down your right leg and stretch out your left side.

♦ With your left side toward the wall turn your torso toward the wall and "walk" your hands along the wall behind you. Hold the position for about 20 seconds and feel the stretch in your waist and upper back. Slowly walk back. Switch to the other side.

QUADRICEPS STRETCHES

♦ Balance yourself against a wall with your left hand. With your right hand grab your left foot behind your back and pull your foot toward your buttocks. Hold it there for about 20 seconds, keeping your knees slightly bent and your back straight. Switch legs.

♦ Assume the "stride position"—one leg forward and vertical to the ground (with the knee over the ankle, not the toes) and the other leg stretched back as far as it can comfortably go. Stretch your groin toward the ground, as if someone behind you is pushing your buttocks down. If your knees hurt, rest your back knee on the ground, with the top of your foot on the ground as well, and push forward with your hands. Lean into the stretch and hold it for about 20 seconds. Switch to the other leg. You should feel the stretch in the quadriceps of your back leg and your groin.

CALF STRETCHES

♦ To stretch the upper calf, stand three feet from a wall. Lean in toward the wall and place your hands on the wall at shoulder height. Step forward with one leg, bending your knee and keeping your foot pointed straight ahead. Straighten your back leg and press your weight on your back foot. Hold the stretch for about 20 seconds. Switch legs.

♦ To stretch the lower calf, again, stand three feet from the wall, lean in toward it, and place your hands on the wall at shoulder height. Step forward with one leg, but this time keep the forward leg straight and bend the back knee. Keeping your heels on the ground and your upper body straight, hold the stretch for 20 seconds. Switch legs.

HAMSTRING STRETCHES

♦ Standing with one leg crossed in front of the other, slowly bend forward, one vertebra at a time, allowing the body to "hang" comfortably. Your knees should be straight but not locked; keep them "'soft." Hold the stretch for 20 seconds and then roll back up slowly. Let your abdominal muscles help you up, not your back. Cross your legs in the other direction and repeat.

♦ Standing with your feet a few inches apart, slowly roll your torso down one vertebra at a time. Hold the stretch for 20 seconds and then roll back up slowly.

GROIN STRETCHES

♦ Sitting with your legs as far apart as you can comfortably stretch them, lean out over one leg and hold a stretch for 20 seconds. Move to the middle, lean over, and hold a stretch for 20 seconds. Then lean to the opposite side for 20 seconds. You'll feel this stretch in your hamstrings as well as your groin.

♦ Sit with your knees bent and the bottoms of your feet together. Bring your heels as close to your groin as you comfortably can. Holding on to your ankles, push down on your knees with your elbows and hold the stretch for 20 seconds.

BUTTOCKS STRETCHES

♦ Sitting on the ground, grab your right ankle and knee and cradle your right leg in your arms. Your left leg may be straight or bent, whichever gives you the best balance. Pull your knee and ankle to your chest and hold the stretch for 20 seconds. Switch to the other leg.

♦ Sit on the floor with your left leg straight out in front of you and your right leg bent. Your right foot should be on the outside of your left knee, and the outside of your right ankle is against the outside of your left knee. Turn your body to the right, placing your left elbow on the outside of your right leg. Now put your right hand on the floor behind you for support and look behind you, pushing against the right leg with your left elbow. Hold the stretch for 20 seconds and switch sides.

TOTAL BODY STRETCH

♦ Stand about an arm's length away from a wall. Step back about a foot and place your feet a couple of inches apart, toes pointing forward. Lean into the wall and walk your hands down the wall to waist height. Keep your back flat. Lock your elbows and knees, and push your tailbone up as far as it will go. Exhale into the stretch and hold it for 20 seconds. To increase the stretch push your tailbone up a little more and drop your chest.

9

Aerobic exercise makes you slim and gives you endurance, stretching exercises make you flexible, but only strength training—also called resistance training or weight training—can make you strong. True fitness combines endurance with flexibility and strength.

People are starting to get the message. A few years ago our Above the Belt, Below the Belt, and Introduction to Weights classes were not exactly high on our guests' lists, but today they're right up there with Low Impact Aerobics and Stretch and Flex. Weight training, once considered the exclusive province of muscle-bound men, is winning new converts of both sexes every day, and for very good reason.

Strength training improves your posture, lets you shape your body as no other exercise can, and makes carrying groceries and shoveling snow a whole lot easier. It can improve your sports performance and protect you from injuries, and it makes your bones dense and strong (a professional tennis player has about 40 percent more bone mass in his playing arm than in the other). Some people like it because of the discipline it demands; others enjoy the control it gives them, as they single out a muscle group and give it increased strength, definition, and shape. Still others, especially women, enjoy the confidence that increased strength brings. To some people the best thing about weight training is the solitude and the quiet.

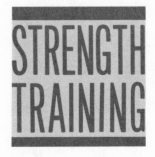

STRENGTH TRAINING

THE TERRIBLE TRUTH ABOUT SPOT REDUCING

There are many misconceptions attached to fitness, but perhaps the most common one has to do with spot reducing, or body contouring, as it's sometimes called. The sad truth is that it can't be done. All the leg lifts in the world won't change the shape of your leg or get rid of saddlebags. You can do abdominal crunches for 12 hours a day, and you won't do anything about a flabby stomach. The body just doesn't work that way.

The only fitness activity that helps you get rid of fat (regardless of where it is) is aerobic exercise, and the only way you can change the shape of and strengthen muscles is through resistance exercise. Before you start thinking that you've wasted the best years of your life in Body Toning class, understand that there is nothing wrong with leg lifts and abdominal crunches; they burn up a few calories and increase your muscular endurance if you do enough of them on a consistent basis. But they do not change the shape of your body. The only thing that can do that is working with weights.

THE PRINCIPLES OF STRENGTH TRAINING

There are two variables in weight training: overload (how much you lift) and repetition (how many times you lift it). The higher the overload is, the fewer repetitions you will be able to do. The goal is, quite simply, to subject a muscle to enough overload so that it becomes fatigued at approximately eight repetitions. Muscular fatigue at eight to ten repetitions is what you need to change the shape of a muscle. If you are able to do more than 12, you're working on muscular endurance, not muscle configuration. So much for doing 50 leg lifts.

The official definition of strength is how much force a muscle can produce in one maximal effort, and it is generally accepted that in training you should lift a weight that's at least 65 percent of your capacity. That number is called your *threshold*. For instance, if you can press 100 pounds, you should be training at 65 pounds or more; that is, doing approximately eight repetitions with 65 or more pounds should fatigue that muscle.

Always start with small weights and work your way up, concentrating on getting your form right. When it becomes easy to do 8 to 12 reps, add a few pounds and start the process again.

MACHINES VERSUS FREE WEIGHTS

If you want to start an argument in a weight room, get people talking about which are better—weight machines or free weights. When the dust settles, you'll be left with a very simple answer. Both develop strength. Both have advantages and disadvantages. The best one is the one you like best and will use consistently.

THE ROMAN CHAIR

If you have back problems, you should approach weight training with extreme caution. The biggest concern among weight trainers is a weak lower back. If you have tight hamstrings, a tight lower back, and weak abdominal muscles in addition to a weak lower back, you may be looking for trouble. Do back exercises regularly; stretches for the hamstrings and lower back and abdominal exercises will help a lot, but one of the best strengtheners specifically for the back is the back extension, which you do on the "Roman Chair." It also can be done quite well on the lower back machine. Anyone with disk problems or nerve damage should see a doctor before doing any back exercises.

Hang your upper body over the end of a bench, with the lower part of your body horizontal. (You can also do this hanging over a bed with someone sitting on your feet.) Lift your upper body until it's parallel to the floor—don't arch your back—and hold the position for two to five seconds. Lower your torso slowly, pause, and come back up again. Do this six to ten times. The Roman Chair is good for the hamstrings and the buttocks as well as the back.

(For more about caring for your back see Chapter 11.)

WEIGHT MACHINES

If there is a line anywhere in your health club or gym, it probably forms at the weight machines. Weight machines are safe, they're easy to use, they do a good job of isolating muscle groups, and people love them. Especially for people just starting out with weight training, machines educate you a little, and they protect you from hurting yourself since your body is virtually locked into place. If you use them properly, they are very effective at developing strength.

Some machines are good for only a single exercise; others—called "multi-station machines"—allow for several different exercises.

There are a few drawbacks to using weight machines. First, since machines are generally too large and too expensive to keep at home, your workout schedule isn't as flexible as it might otherwise be. Second, there are those lines. Some health clubs want you to do your 8 to 12 reps and move on; they don't take kindly to people who come back for second and third sets. And finally, if you get really serious about your training, machines might not give you enough variety.

FREE WEIGHTS

Free weights, the generic term for what used to be called dumbbells and barbells, have several obvious advantages: they're cheap, they're portable, they improve balance and coordination in addition to making you stronger, and they are extremely versatile. A starter set of weights (5-, 8-, 10-, and 20-pound weights) will cost you about 50 dollars. Even a bench press, which is considered by many to be the perfect weight training tool, is not too expensive.

Most weight training purists feel that free weights give them more control of their lifting than machines and more discipline as well. In a way weight machines do much of the thinking for you, which is why so many people like them. With free weights you are completely in charge, and the technique requires a relatively high level of concentration. The other side of that coin is that all that freedom and creativity make users of free weights slightly more injury-prone than people who use machines.

The Push-Up

For people who like to build their muscles the old-fashioned way the push-up is still one of the best resistance exercises there is. (In this case, of course, it's your body weight that offers the resistance.) Push-ups work the muscles in the shoulders, the upper arms, and the chest, and they also exercise muscles in the abdomen. But you have to do them right.

THE STANDARD PUSH-UP
Lie face down on the ground and place the palms of your hands on the floor slightly wider than shoulder width just outside your chest. Keeping your feet close together and your knees locked, straighten your arms. From shoulder to ankles your body should be in a straight line throughout the exercise. Push yourself up slowly, without sagging in the middle. Lower yourself slowly, touching your chest to the floor for a second but not resting. Breathe evenly, exhaling as you go up and inhaling on the way down.

MODIFIED PUSH-UPS
If you're not yet strong enough for a standard push-up, start with a modified version and work up to it. One way to make it a little easier is to pivot from your knees instead of your feet. Be sure that you keep your torso completely straight; it's a common mistake to arch your back and let your abdomen sag.

Another modified version of the push-up is the "let-down," an exercise based on the premise that it's easier to hold your body up than it is to lift it. Start in the "up" position of a standard push-up and slowly lower your body until your chest is just about on the floor, again keeping your back in a straight line. Then, using your knees, return to the "up" position. Once the let-down becomes easy, you can graduate to the push-up.

THE ADVANCED VERSION

To work the triceps even more place your hands close together on the floor and flare out your elbows. To work the chest more place your hands farther apart. To increase the weight you're lifting put your feet on a chair, bench, or step as you do standard push-ups. The incline forces you to use the muscles in your upper chest as well as your shoulders and triceps.

GETTING STARTED

If you'd like to start a weight training program, it's a good idea to get someone who knows the ropes of weight training to show you how it's done and supervise you, at least for the first few sessions. Whether you use machines or free weights or a combination of the two, form is critical. Crowded weight rooms are not the perfect spot to take Weight Training 101, so you may want to arrange for a private session or two until you gain some confidence.

Here are some of the basics to keep in mind:

♦ Consider your weight. If you're very overweight, you would do well to get rid of the fat layer—through diet and aerobic exercise—before you embark on a weight training program. Once you get within ten pounds or so of your goal weight, it will be easier to see results.

♦ Warm up before you lift. Think of your muscles as Turkish taffy. When taffy is cold, it snaps and tears; when it's warm, it stretches. Before you start your workout spend five continuous minutes walking briskly, cycling, running in place, rowing, or skipping rope. You can also do a light set, of 10 or 12 repetitions, of the exercises you are planning to do.

♦ Watch your form. More than any other kind of exercise weight training requires precision. You can pretty much do aerobic exercises any which way, as long as your heart rate stays up and you don't injure yourself, but that's not so with weights. Speed doesn't count here. Strive for smooth, controlled movements during both the lifting and the let-down phases. If you're having trouble doing it right, you may be trying to lift too much or using the wrong muscles. Start out slowly. Even if it seems too easy at first, start with very low weights until you have perfected your technique. Then increase the resistance.

♦ Don't forget to breathe. If a crowd starts to gather around you, and people begin asking if you're okay, chances are you've been holding your breath when you lift. Remember, exhale on exertion.

♦ Keep things in balance. As strange as it sounds, lots of people work on only one side of their bodies—bench presses, curls, abdominals, and that's it. As a result they develop the front portion of their body, but they don't have any upper back or leg development at all. If you get really strong on one side of your body, the chances of injury to the weak side become greater, and you may develop a peculiar shape.

♦ Don't worry about bulking up. This is not bodybuilding. The sort of strength training we are talking about here develops the muscles and gives them better shape and give you modest increases in strength. You are in control of how far you want to progress. When you reach your goal, don't continue to increase the weights. Start a maintenance program.

♦ Stretch afterward. When you're finished with the session and your muscles are still warm, spend five or ten minutes stretching each muscle group of the body. Hold each stretch statically (don't bounce) for 20 to 30 seconds.

♦ Don't overdo it. Be sure you rest for 48 hours between weight training workouts. On your off-days do aerobics or stretching exercises.

♦ Don't expect immediate results. Even if you lift for 30 minutes at a time three times a week, it will probably be about two months before you really notice a change in your body. It may take even longer for women, because their testosterone level, which aids in developing muscles, is lower than men's.

THE CANYON RANCH TAKE-HOME STRENGTH PROGRAM

The take-home strength program that we offer our guests was devised by exercise physiologist Denise Gater, one of the most enthusiastic supporters that strength training ever had. (The two staunchest proponents of weight training at the Ranch are women; Meredith Wittwer is the other.) The workout includes five different exercises with free weights and a short workout series for the abdominals and lower back. Each exercise is designed to use as many muscle groups as possible, so you can use your time efficiently. The complete workout takes about 30 minutes, including the warm-up and the post-workout stretching.

You'll need access to a little equipment: a flat bench, two adjustable dumbbells, and a belt or strap to hold your legs down for back extensions. The weight you lift should be heavy enough so that muscular failure (that's what it's called when a muscle is too tired to continue) is reached at the specified number of repetitions. Do not sacrifice form for heavier weight.

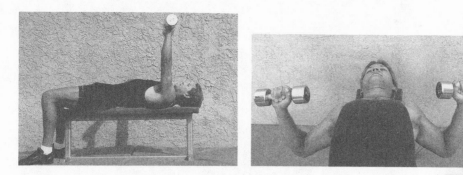

Lie flat on your back, feet flat on the floor with buttocks, upper back and head in contact with the bench throughout the entire exercise. Start by lifting dumbbells so that they are directly over the shoulder joints with elbows straight, and dumbbell heads touching (Figure 1). Slowly lower the dumbbells as far as possible to the side of the torso, so that the dumbbells are in line with the chest and you feel a stretch in this area. The upper and lower arm should make a 90 degree angle at the elbow in this bottom position (Figure 2). As you press the dumbbells upward, they should move from your chest in a slightly concave fashion (curving toward your head) so that they end up directly over the shoulder joints once again, dumbbell heads touching at the top (Figure 1).

Alternate Dumbbell Bench Presses with Single Arm Rows

DUMBBELL BENCH PRESS

MAJOR MUSCLE GROUPS:

Pectoralis Major (chest) Anterior Deltoid (front of shoulder) Triceps (back of upper arm)

SINGLE ARM ROWS

MAJOR MUSCLE GROUPS:

Latissimus Dorsi (upper back) Posterior Deltoid (back of shoulder) Elbow Flexors (front of upper and lower arm)

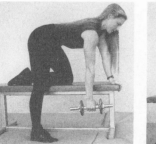
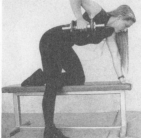

For lower back support, place left hand, with elbow extended but not in a locked position, and left knee on a flat bench. Keep shoulders as parallel to the floor as possible throughout the entire exercise. Start with the dumbbell in right hand directly under right shoulder, with elbow extended and palm facing in (Figure 3). Lift elbow up toward the ceiling, keeping dumbbell close to the ribs with shoulder down and the torso as stationary as possible (Figure 4). Slowly lower dumbbell back to starting position (Figure 3). Repeat exercise with left arm.

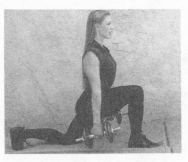

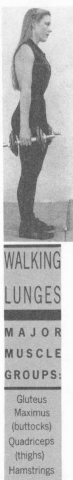

WALKING
LUNGES

MAJOR
MUSCLE
GROUPS:

Gluteus
Maximus
(buttocks)
Quadriceps
(thighs)
Hamstrings
(back of thigh)

After several workouts using only body weight, this exercise can be done with dumbbells as shown here. From the starting position (Figure 5) take a large step forward so that the front knee is directly over the ankle (Figure 6). Be sure not to let the knee go beyond the toes. Keep head and chest up throughout the entire movement. Back knee may bend depending upon flexibility. Push up and back off front leg and bring the back leg forward until you are standing upright. Prepare for the next step with the opposite leg. Go down slowly and up fast. This is an excellent exercise to do up a ramp or hill if weights are not available, or as a variation.

Alternate Walking Lunges with Dumbbell Overhead Presses and Dumbbell Curls.

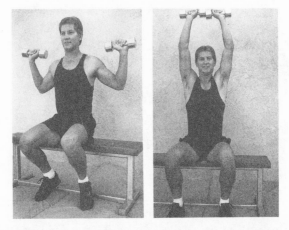

DUMBBELL
OVERHEAD
PRESS

MAJOR
MUSCLE
GROUPS:

Deltoid (shoulder)
Triceps (back of
upper arm)
Trapezius (upper
middle back)

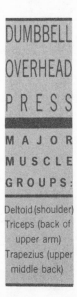

Sit on an upright or flat bench. Take an overhand grip on dumbbells with hands slightly wider than shoulder width apart and forearms nearly perpendicular to the floor (Figure 7). Keep back flat as you press the dumbbells upward, extending elbows over head until dumbbell heads touch at the top (Figure 8). Let dumbbells down slowly to starting position.

DUMBBELL CURLS

MAJOR MUSCLE GROUPS:

Biceps (front of upper arm)

Place feet 12 inches from a wall. Slightly bend knees and press lower and upper back flat against the wall. With palms up, hold dumbbell heads together with elbows extended such that the dumbbells are touching the quadriceps, or thighs (Figure 9). Without moving anything but the elbow joint, lift dumbbells toward the clavicles, or collar bone (Figure 10). Do not swing dumbbells or arch back to lift heavier weights. Slowly lower dumbbells until elbows are extended back into the starting position, touching the quadriceps (Figure 9).

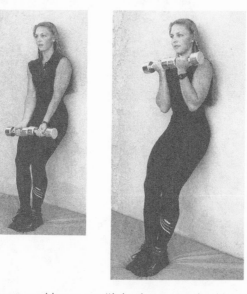

BACK EXTENSIONS

MAJOR MUSCLE GROUPS:

Spinal Erectors (lower back)
Gluteus Maximus (buttocks)
Hamstrings (back of thigh)

Individuals with disk or nerve problems, or with back spasms should *not* do this exercise. This should not be a fast, jerky exercise, but a slow, controlled movement. Place a belt or strap around a flat bench to hold your ankles down. Start with hips flexed as much as possible (Figure 15). With a flat back, and hands in front of forehead, extend hips until body is horizontal with the floor (Figure 16). Do NOT arch back at the top. Slowly return to starting position.

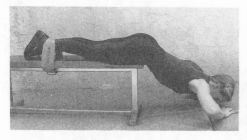
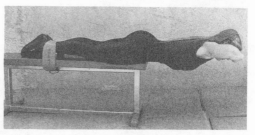

ABDOMINAL CRUNCH SERIES

MAJOR MUSCLE GROUPS:

Rectus Abdominis (abdominal muscles)
Obliques (waist)

The following four exercises should be done in order. Do ten repetitions of each exercise (one set) before resting.

1. Crunches with a Pelvic Tilt

Interlace fingers behind head at base of neck. Focus eyes on ceiling throughout the exercise. With lower back in contact with the floor and lower legs on flat bench, flex trunk into the "crunch" position while simultaneously doing a pelvic tilt with the pelvis (Figure 11). Hold five seconds in this "crunch" position. Return upper back and pelvis to the floor slowly, and immediately start the next repetition without resting.

2. Twisting Crunches

With the lower back in contact with the floor and lower legs on flat bench, flex and twist trunk lifting shoulders off the floor with elbow headed towards opposite knee (Figure 12). Slowly return upper back and shoulders to floor. On the next repetition, twist in the other direction.

3. Fast Crunches with Legs Up

Begin exercise with legs up, knee and hip joints at 90 degrees, calves parallel to the floor. Flex trunk into the "crunch" position, while bringing knees and elbows together until they touch (Figure 13). Slowly return upper back to the floor.

4. Bicycles

With the lower back in contact with the floor, alternate elbow to opposite knee (Figure 14) rotating at the waist as much as possible. Keep knees bent throughout the exercise.

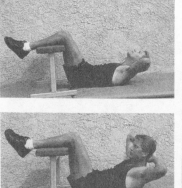
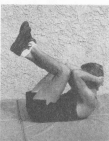
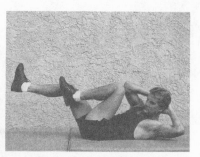

10

Don't slouch!" To anyone who's ever had a mother or a third-grade teacher, that command probably has an all-too-familiar ring to it. Well, your mother and your teacher weren't right about everything they told you to do when you were a kid, but they were right about that.

Chances are, however, that they were scolding you because they thought you looked terrible all slumped over like that. What they may not have known is that proper posture is also vital to the way you feel. Bad posture when you sit or stand makes you achy and tired, and it can cause back and neck aches, sciatica, foot problems, even disk damage. You can end up with lower back pain, headaches, and upper body tension. Bad posture can even make you grind your teeth. Besides, you do look terrible all slumped over like that!

Are you the kind of person who feels great on Monday but tired and achy and out of sorts by the time the weekend rolls around? It could very well be because you've been sitting all week, leaning forward over your papers, or balancing the phone between your chin and shoulder for hours without a break. Standing exerts five times more pressure on the back than lying down, and sitting at a desk is even harder on the back. Worse still is sitting behind the wheel of your car. It's no wonder you can't wait until Friday.

How Do You Rate?

Look at your profile in a full-length mirror. You'll probably see a protruding abdomen, slumped or rounded shoulders, perhaps even a swayback. Now drop your shoulders and relax them and begin "lift-off." Lift your head (keep

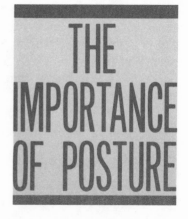

THE
IMPORTANCE
OF POSTURE

your chin level). Next lift your ribs off your waist and your waist up off your hips. Now, keeping your tailbone down, lift your entire body weight up, as if a string attached to the crown of your head is being pulled tight to the ceiling. Congratulations! You now have perfect posture. If only it were that easy.

A Posture Inventory, Head to Toe

At the Ranch one of the "awareness services" we perform is a posture analysis, during which we closely examine a guest's posture and make recommendations about how various improvements can be made. We also take "before" and "after" pictures so that our guests can see what a remarkable difference even small changes in posture can make in their appearance. We suggest that you do the same at home. Here are the specific areas we examine and "grade" in our sessions and the common problems we find.

♦ Your head should be straight up. Common problem: it may twist slightly or even markedly to one side.

♦ Your shoulders should be level. Common problem: one may be higher than the other.

♦ Your spine should be straight. Common problem: it may be curved laterally.

♦ Your hips should be level. Common problem: one may be higher than the other.

♦ Your ankles should be straight. Common problem: if your feet point outward instead of straight ahead, your ankles will sag.

♦ Your neck should be erect, holding your head in balance directly above your shoulders. Common problem: many people keep the neck forward with the chin out.

♦ Your upper back should be only slightly rounded. Common problem: it may be more rounded than it should be.

♦ Your trunk should be erect. Common problem: it may tilt back to the rear.

♦ Your abdomen should be flat. Common problem: it may protrude and sag.

♦ Your lower back should curve slightly. Common problem: it may be more hollow than curved.

NAME _____

	GOOD—10	FAIR—5	POOR—0	SCORING DATES		
HEAD LEFT RIGHT	Head erect gravity line passes directly through center	Head twisted or turned to one side slightly	Head twisted or turned to one side markedly			
SHOULDERS LEFT RIGHT	Shoulders level (horizontally)	One shoulder slightly higher than other	One shoulder markedly higher than other			
SPINE LEFT RIGHT	Spine straight	Spine slightly curved laterally	Spine markedly curved laterally			
HIPS LEFT RIGHT	Hips level (horizontally)	One hip slightly higher	One hip markedly higher			
ANKLES	Feet pointed straight ahead	Feet pointed out	Feet pointed out markedly; ankles sag in (Pronation)			
NECK	Neck erect, chin in, head in balance directly above shoulders	Neck slightly forward, chin slightly out	Neck markedly forward, chin markedly out			
UPPER BACK	Upper back normally rounded	Upper back slightly more rounded	Upper back markedly rounded			
TRUNK	Trunk erect	Trunk inclined to rear slightly	Trunk inclined to rear markedly			
ABDOMEN	Abdomen flat	Abdomen protruding	Abdomen protruding and sagging			
LOWER BACK	Lower back normally curved	Lower back slightly hollow	Lower back markedly hollow			
			TOTAL SCORES			

How to Fix It

Now that you have some idea of what you're doing wrong, what can you do about it? There are several things, but the first and most important one is to decide you're going to change. The way we stand and sit and carry packages and talk on the phone is a habit, and like any other habitual behavior, it can be changed. You just have to want to change and to know how. If you're heavier than you should be, think about losing weight. The more overweight you are, the harder it is for you to maintain correct posture. After all, what you do when you stand and sit up straight is fight gravity. Gravity pulls you down, and the most important word in good posture is "up."

Regardless of your weight, the following tips should work wonders for your posture. Some of them may seem awkward at first—more than one of our guests has said it's a lot like patting your head and rubbing your stomach at the same time—but after a few practice sessions the new ways will begin to feel more natural. Eventually good posture will be automatic.

TIPS FOR STANDING

♦ Keep your head up and your chin in.
♦ Lift your body from the breastbone.
♦ Relax your shoulders and keep them level.
♦ Pull your abdomen in tight. Draw it in and up.
♦ Keep your hips level.
♦ Tilt your pelvis forward slightly.
♦ Flex your buttocks muscles.
♦ Keep your feet parallel, with your weight evenly distributed.
♦ Straighten your spine.

Special tip: If you're on your feet all day, take the pressure off your spine whenever you can by resting a foot on a low stool or railing. Alternate feet regularly.

TIPS FOR SITTING

♦ Keep your chin in.
♦ Sit straight up in your chair, with your spine lifted from the head and chest. Don't lean back; your upper back should not be pressed against the chair.
♦ Your lower back should touch the chair. A slight curve in the lower back is natural and desirable. If necessary, put a towel or sweater behind you to maintain the curve.
♦ Keep your feet flat on the floor. Don't cross your legs.
♦ Lean forward slightly—from the hips, not from the waist.

Special tip: To stretch and relax your muscles during desk work, reach around behind you and clasp your hands together behind the chair. (If you can't reach, stretch as far as you can.) Hold the position for a minute or two.

TIPS FOR WALKING

♦ Start by standing correctly. Be sure your body stays aligned properly as you walk.

♦ Keep your feet parallel.

♦ Use a rolling motion, landing on the heel and rolling to the ball of the foot.

♦ Move freely and rhythmically. Don't tense up.

THREE MORE POSTURE TIPS

♦ Automobile seats are murder on your back; ask anyone who spends a lot of time out on the road. When you're driving, move your car seat forward so that your knees are bent. A small pillow placed at your lower back can help to maintain a slight curve in your lower back. When you have to spend hours in a car, get out regularly and stretch.

♦ When you're carrying something heavy, don't arch your lower back or twist your body. Maintain proper body alignment and let your arms and abdominal muscles carry the weight.

♦ Even sleeping can create back problems, particularly if you're used to sleeping on your stomach. Train yourself to sleep on your side with your knees bent. Get yourself a firm mattress.

POSTURE EXERCISES

Moving your body on a regular basis is good for virtually anything that ails you. Posture is no exception. Aerobic exercise is recommended because it helps you keep your weight down, and stretching is good because it keeps you loose. However, the most helpful exercise for promoting good posture is strength training; the stronger your muscles are, the more easily they can support your skeletal system, which is what good posture is all about. Concentrate on weight training that strengthens the pectoral area and the upper back muscles.

Here are a few specific exercises:

♦ Sitting or standing with your hands behind your head, press your head back into your hands while keeping your elbows parallel. Hold the position for ten seconds. Repeat five times.

♦ Sitting or standing with your hands behind your head, lower your chin to your chest, keeping your back nice and tall. Touch your elbows together and hold the position for ten seconds. Slowly roll your head up, one vertebra at a time, keeping your elbows open. Repeat five times.

♦ Stand facing a corner with your feet together, keeping your sternum lifted and your buttocks contracted. Bring your chest toward the corner, keeping your body lifted, and return to the standing position. Repeat five times.

♦ Clasp your hands behind your back. Keeping your knees bent, your chest lifted, and your pubic bone forward, rest the back of your thumbs against your tailbone. Breathe in and out slowly, pressing your elbows together and keeping your sternum tall. Repeat five times.

PRACTICE MAKES PERFECT

If we said that perfect posture comes naturally, we'd be lying. In fact, all of this may feel very strange indeed, at least at first. Our muscles have an excellent memory, and getting them to forget what they've been doing for a lot of years takes time. No, we can't promise that it will be easy, but we can promise that it feels great once you've trained yourself to do it. Eventually standing tall and sitting up straight will be a reflex; the old way will start to make you feel uncomfortable. First, though, there's the practice, and that string attached to the top of your head.

Working on your posture may make you feel self-conscious—many women feel funny about lifting their chests out—but if you need any encouragement, take a quick look at those "before" and "after" pictures you took earlier and think about which you would rather be. Remember that even a small change can make a huge difference. And don't slouch!

11

Sooner or later, just about everyone has back trouble, and it's no wonder. Between bad posture, excess weight, lack of exercise, sudden wrong moves, and a cavalier attitude about heavy lifting, our backs take a terrific beating. For some people this will mean occasional twinges. For others it will be something more serious, such as disk problems or arthritis. For most it's something in between, such as chronic lower back pain.

There are almost as many theories about how to relieve back pain as there are cures for hiccups. Everyone gets into the act—doctors, osteopaths, chiropractors, orthopedists, physical therapists, aunts, uncles, and the guys at the office—and some of their cures even work. What works best with backs, though, is prevention.

How to Baby Your Back

You've been walking, standing, and dressing yourself for quite a while now, and you probably think you have the rudiments down pat. However, as you'll quickly discover if and when your back starts bothering you, you can't take even the most elementary move for granted. You may have to learn how to move all over again. Try doing it like this.

♦ Standing. Avoid prolonged standing whenever possible. If you must stand in one place for a prolonged period of time, occasionally rest one foot on a low footstool or small box. As you do so, flex your knees and hips and flatten your lower back.

♦ Sitting. Sit all the way back in your chair with your back erect and your knees bent. If

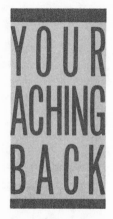

YOUR ACHING BACK

possible, elevate your knees higher than your hips.

♦ Driving. Keep your seat close to the steering wheel to elevate the knees. On long trips stop every hour or two to stretch and relax your muscles.

♦ Walking. A heel-toe rolling motion is best; land on your heel and push off on the ball of your foot. Avoid high heels.

♦ Bending. Always bend at the knees, with your buttocks tucked under you.

♦ Sleeping. The ideal position is curled up on your side with your knees bent. The worst for your back is sleeping on your stomach. If you choose to compromise and sleep on your back, putting a pillow under your knees will keep your lower back flat.

♦ Lifting. Avoid unnecessary reaching and lifting. When you do pick things up off the floor, bend at the hips and knees, not the waist, and keep your back rounded as you return to a standing position. Always face your work and turn by pivoting your feet first.

♦ Dressing. Sit down to dress. Don't bend from the waist while trying to balance on one foot.

Choosing the Right Sport

On the one hand, exercise is great for your back; it makes you strong, and it can help to eliminate the pot belly that's weighing you down. On the other hand, exercise can be murder on the back if it's the wrong kind. In general people with back trouble should avoid exercises that strain the back or arch it excessively. High-risk sports are any that involve lifting, twisting, arching of the spine, sudden starts and stops, falls, and collisions with other players. Of course, even the lowest-risk sport can be bad for you if you do too much too soon, and a high-risk sport can be made acceptable if you're careful.

"good" sports

If you have back problems, these are the best fitness activities for you.

♦ Walking. Walking puts less strain on the spine than unsupported sitting and only a little more than standing. In terms of back comfort, it's virtually a perfect exercise, provided you wear the right shoes and stay away from very steep hills.

♦ Swimming. This is a great exercise too, since the water supports your spine, relieving pressure. The breast stroke and butterfly tend to make you arch your back, so avoid them if your back actually hurts. Much better are the crawl, the side stroke, and, appropriately enough, the back stroke. Using a snorkel may reduce back strain.

♦ Jogging. If you do it right, jogging can be perfectly acceptable. Be sure to run on soft surfaces in well-cushioned shoes and practice a smooth stride.

♦ Cycling. Provided you remain upright, you shouldn't have any problems.

♦ Rowing. Form is critical here. If you do it right, it can strengthen the back; if you do it wrong, it will make matters worse. Always keep your back straight. Don't hunch over or sway as you row.

"BAD" SPORTS

These activities may well make a bad back worse:

♦ Golf. Twenty-five percent of all golf pros suffer from lower back injuries, and it's not hard to imagine why. Golf involves all sorts of motions that can strain the spine: teeing the ball, removing the ball from the cup, and, of course, the twisting movement of the swing itself. You can lessen the risk by always bending at the knees with your back straight and swinging with a minimum of twist.

♦ Tennis and other racquet sports. The sudden stops and starts and twists of most racquet sports often lead to back strain. If you're having trouble, consider modifying your serve and your backhand, which are particularly rough on the spine.

♦ Bowling. Want back trouble? Try lifting a heavy weight while twisting and bending your upper body. Using a light ball and practicing a smooth delivery can minimize risk.

♦ Football, basketball, and baseball. Professional athletes don't quit in their twenties and thirties because they get bored. All that twisting, jarring, jumping, bending, not to mention serious contact with other players, is murder on the spine.

♦ Weightlifting. Lifting some weights puts a great deal of stress on the lower back; if you have serious back trouble, you would be wise to avoid weightlifting until you get stronger. Form is critical to safe weightlifting. (See Chapter 9.) When you pick up something heavy—whether it's a toddler or a bag of groceries or a barbell—keep the back straight and let your legs help lift by bending your knees.

EXERCISES TO STRENGTHEN THE BACK

One of the best ways to avoid back injury is to keep the back supple and strengthen the stomach and back muscles. Here are some specific exercises that should help.

♦ Bent leg sit-up. Lie on your back with your knees bent and your feet flat up on a chair or table. Fold your arms across your chest and tuck your chin close into your chest. Contract your abdominals and slowly raise your trunk about eight inches off the floor and hold the position for five seconds. Slowly roll your spine to the floor, one vertebra at a time. Repeat the exercise ten times.

♦ Pelvic tilt. Lie on your back with your knees bent and your feet flat on the floor. Flatten your lower back and press it to the floor. Tighten your abdominal muscles and buttocks and tilt your pelvis upward, putting weight on your heels. Hold the position for five counts, making sure to breathe. Relax and return your hips to the floor. Repeat ten times.

♦ Upper back strengthener. Roll onto your abdomen and place a pillow under your waist. Lie with your forehead down and arms stretched out at your sides. Lift your head, shoulders, and arms off the floor. Hold for five counts and relax. Repeat five times.

♦ Lower back stretch. Lie on your back with your legs out straight in front of you. Grasp your right knee with both hands and pull it toward your chin, keeping the other leg straight. (Pull it as far as it will go without causing pain.) Hold it for five counts and release your leg slowly to the floor. Repeat with the left leg and then with both legs at the same time. Repeat the series five times.

♦ Lower back strengthener. Lie on your abdomen with your arms folded under your head. Keeping both hip bones flat on the floor, tighten the buttocks and elevate one leg slightly without bending your knee. (You may want to put a pillow under your waist.) Hold for five seconds and slowly lower your leg to the floor. Change to the other leg. Repeat five times with each leg.

♦ Mad Cat/Saggy Horse. Get down on all fours. Press your chin toward your chest and arch your back. Hold it for five seconds. Then slowly allow your head to come up as you release your abdominal muscles and drop your back down. Repeat five times.

♦ Prayer position. Get down on all fours. Move forward along the floor onto your forearms, keeping your back and neck straight. Lower your buttocks onto your heels, place your forehead on the floor, and continue the stretch. Relax in this position for 15 seconds.

PAINS IN THE NECK

Where there is back trouble, there is likely to be neck trouble, and vice versa. Here are a few ways to save your neck.

DON'T:

♦ Read in bed with your head propped up high or watch television in bed.

♦ Sleep with a large pillow.

♦ Sleep on your stomach. Train yourself to sleep on your back or, preferably, your side.

♦ Put your car seat too low or too far back from the wheel when you're driving.

♦ Stretch for objects out of easy reach. Use a stool. Tilt your head back when you're at the movies. Unless you're sitting in the front row, this isn't usually necessary, but it's a common habit.

♦ Fall asleep in a chair. It's no wonder most of us are a wreck after trying to sleep on a plane.

DO:

♦ Sleep with your arms at your side.

♦ When you sit in a chair, lean forward from the hips (not your waist) and keep your chin in close.

♦ Experiment with your pillow so that your head and neck are in a "neutral" position.

♦ Use your arms to lift yourself out of a chair or a car. Don't thrust your head forward to get leverage.

THE RIGHT CHAIR

Ideally we'd all have an active lifestyle, but the fact is many of us spend our lives in a chair. The least we can do is make it the right, or "ergonomically sound," chair. Sitting can be incredibly stressful to the back; sitting with an unsupported back puts 40 percent more pressure on your spine than standing does. Sitting can be rough on the legs too, particularly if you have circulatory problems. (When you sit, the leg muscles don't contract to pump blood to the heart. Blood pools in the legs, and pressure builds.) Finally, your shoulder and neck muscles take a beating too, as you hunch over a desk or balance a telephone between ear and shoulder for 40 or more hours a week.

The right chair can make your life a lot easier. Look for one that's adjustable every which way; there should be levers for adjusting both the seat height and the angle of the back, and it should also have casters for easy mobility. Look for armrests too, and room enough so that you can shift your weight around easily. The back rest should follow the natural curve of your spine, and the seat should be firm with rounded edges. Finally, look for a five-blade pedestal; it's considerably more stable than one with four.

If you can't buy a brand-new chair, there are ways to improve the lemon you have. Go to a store that sells orthopedic paraphernalia and ask for a lower-back cushion and a seat wedge. The cushion goes behind you and supports the natural curve of your spine. The wedge goes under you and tilts your pelvis forward slightly. As a final touch, put a footstool or a hefty phone book on the floor, and rest your feet on it to take the pressure off your spine. It may not be ergonomically sound, but it's better than nothing.

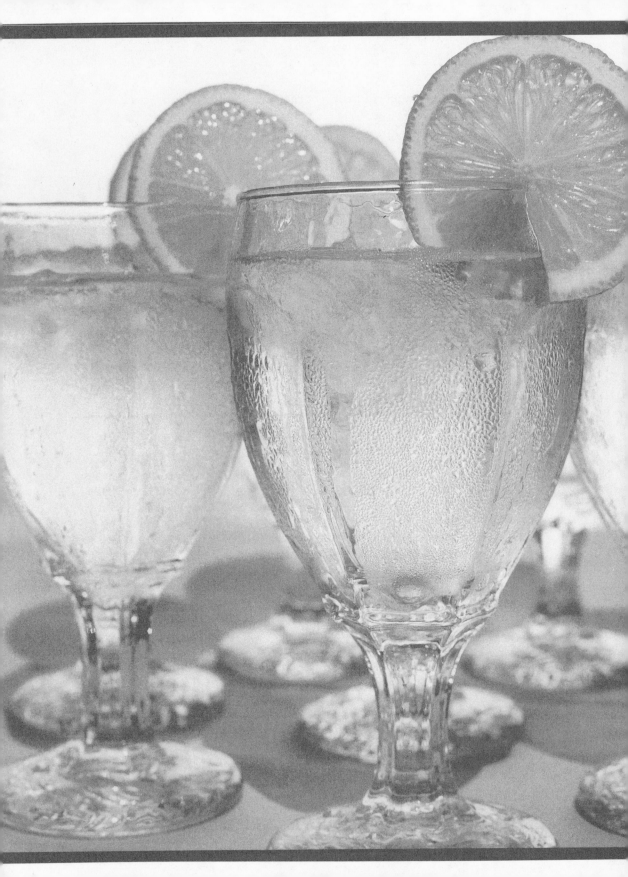

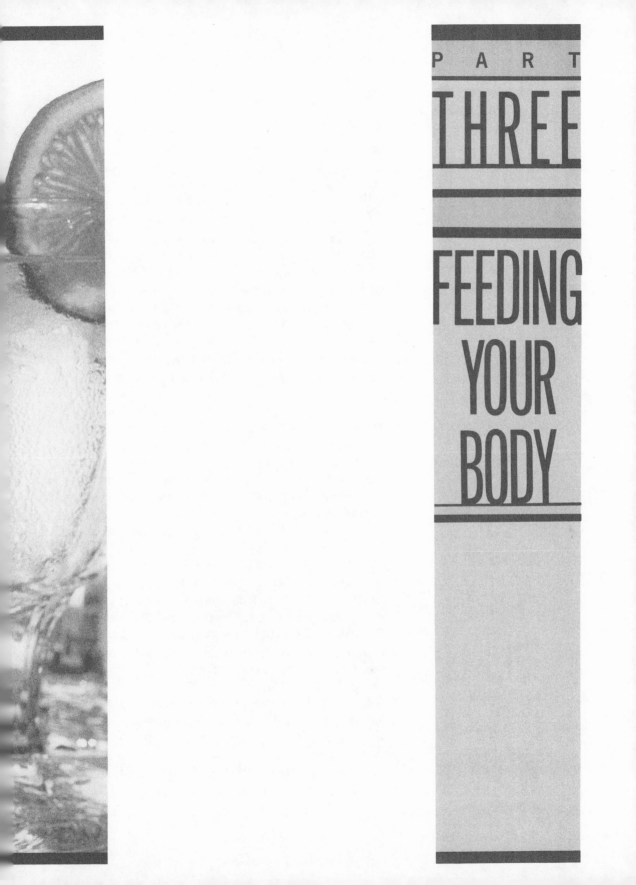

PART

THREE

FEEDING YOUR BODY

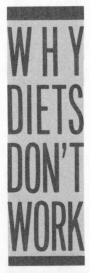

12

WHY DIETS DON'T WORK

Every Monday morning it's the same thing. You wake up, and the first thing that pops into your mind is that you've *got* to do something about your weight. You can't figure out what happened last week; on Monday you were filled with resolve and didn't give dessert a second thought, but by Friday your willpower was almost gone. The weekend was a complete disaster. Now you're lying in bed wondering if it hurts to have your stomach stapled or whether you can talk on the phone if your mouth is taped shut. Visions of liposuction and tummy tucks dance in your head. In short, you're back on a diet.

You're not the only one whose slogan is, "If it's Monday, I must be dieting." According to a 1986 Gallup poll, some 31 percent of American women from age 19 to 39 diet at least once a month. Sixteen percent say they're on diets all the time. We spend about $200 million a year on appetite suppressants.

You would think that all this dieting would have turned us into a nation of wraiths, but of course, it's not so; the United States population is the world's fattest. Obesity is a major public health problem in this country. Two out of five adults are overweight. According to the American Dietetic Association, the average married American woman has gained 23 pounds by her thirteenth wedding anniversary, and her husband has put on 18 pounds.

It is widely known that being overweight is bad for your health. Obesity contributes to hypertension, heart disease, strokes, diabetes, arthritis, gallstones, respiratory disease, and some types of cancer. Yet even in the face of all the persuasive evidence, we can't seem to get rid of those 15 extra pounds. Why is that?

BORN TO BE FAT?

In February of 1988 millions of people picked up their morning papers and learned something that they had suspected all along: some people gain weight more easily and have a bigger problem taking it off than other people. According to recent research, many fat people are actually biochemically different from thin people; their slower metabolic rate (they may burn 20 to 30 percent fewer calories than thin people) makes it extremely difficult to lose or even maintain weight.

The truth was out: to be fat is not necessarily to be lazy or weak or greedy or self-indulgent. Obese people are born with a handicap, and obesity is a disease. However, unlike many diseases, it has a remedy: a safe, sensible approach to fueling the body.

THE PHYSIOLOGY OF WEIGHT LOSS

One of the things we like to do most at the Ranch is teach, and one of our favorite subjects is how food is used by the body. It's always gratifying to see the light bulb go on over a guest's head when he finally realizes why he hasn't been able to get rid of those last ten pounds; why it makes more sense to eat a little more and exercise a little more than to starve himself slim; or why losing more than a couple of pounds a week is asking for trouble. The first step in appreciating all of that is understanding how metabolism works.

THE BASAL METABOLIC RATE

Your basal metabolic rate, or BMR, is the number of calories you need per day to maintain your basic body functions when your body is at rest. For most people that number falls somewhere between, 1000 and 1400 calories. Basically a BMR is born, not made, but there are several factors that affect it:

♦ Age. As you get older, your BMR decreases. Most research indicates a 3 percent drop per decade after age 25.

♦ Gender. Unlike fat, lean mass is metabolically active. Because men have more lean body mass (especially muscles) than women do, they have a higher BMR than women.

♦ Height. The taller you are, the higher your BMR is.

♦ Weight. The more you weigh, the higher your BMR is. For every pound you lose you will burn at least ten calories fewer a day just because you're lighter.

♦ Activity. As we discuss below, your BMR may be increased with vigorous exercise.

EATING TOO LITTLE

Because your body cares more about staying alive than looking good in a bathing suit, when you consume fewer calories than you need to sustain your BMR, your body reacts by going into its "self-preservation" mode, lowering your BMR and conserving calories to protect itself from starvation. This process doesn't necessarily take long, either; in one day, a lowering of calories can reduce your BMR by 10 percent. If you cut your calories less dramatically—to no lower than your basal metabolic rate—your body will continue to operate efficiently as you lose weight.

As strange as it seems, if you eat too few calories, you slow down the weight loss process; sometimes you have to consume a few more calories to lose weight. At the Ranch we recommend a minimum of 1000 calories a day for women and 1200 for men, but 1200 and 1500, respectively, are probably better minimum calorie counts for a long-range weight loss program. Most experts agree that a diet of 1200 calories a day is enough to conserve lean body mass while burning fat, provided you get enough protein and you exercise regularly.

Calorie requirements are different for everyone (and extremely dependent on how much exercise you get), but as a general rule, multiplying your weight by ten gives you a rough estimate of the number of calories you need every day to lose a pound a week.

YO-YO DIETING

A couple of years ago a study was done with overweight laboratory rats who went on a diet and then resumed their regular eating habits. The first time the rats lost their excess weight in 21 days and regained it in 45. The second time around they took 46 days to get the extra weight off and only 14 to gain it all back. Does this scenario sound familiar?

Let's follow what we've talked about so far to its logical conclusion. You go on a crash diet, and your body starts to conserve calories to keep from starving, lowering your BMR and perhaps even depleting muscle mass. Then you go back to your normal eating patterns, and your body, which has become more "efficient" at using fuel sources, packs the pounds back on. Regained weight is especially stubborn. Each time you go on a diet and play games with your BMR, the situation gets worse; weight is harder to lose and easier to gain. What's more, pounds lost as muscle are often regained as fat. What you end up with is a kind of diet-induced obesity.

Chronic dieting is not just tough on the body; seeing your weight go up and down and up again is bad for the head as well.

Yo-yo dieting is clearly not the answer to your weight problem. Here are a few strategies that do work.

In a University of Arizona study a group of obese women in their thirties were divided into three sub-groups: (1) diet, (2) exercise, and (3) diet and exercise. The diet group consumed 700 calories a day and did not exercise. The exercise group ate 1,200 calories per day and used up 500 calories a day in exercise. The diet and exercise group was allowed 950 calories a day and worked off 250 with exercise. After 12 weeks all the groups had lost weight: diet, 11.7 pounds; exercise, 10.6 pounds; diet and exercise, 12 pounds. Pretty close, you're probably thinking, but you're wrong. Weight loss is only part of the story.

The rest of the story was told not by the scale but by the body-fat composition tests of the participants, which measured how much of the weight lost was fat weight and how much was lean weight (muscle, bone, ligaments, tendons, organs, and water). The dieters lost 9.3 pounds of fat weight; the exercisers lost 12.6 pounds of fat; and the dieter/exercisers lost 13 pounds of fat. As you can tell, two of the groups actually gained lean weight. The wild card in weight loss is clearly exercise, specifically aerobic (fat-burning) exercise. It not only burns calories; it also increases your BMR.

Obviously, the weight loss method of choice should be the combination diet-and-exercise route. The best way to lose a pound, or 3500 calories, a week is to lose 500 calories a day, and the best way to do that is to eat 250 calories fewer (one candy bar) and burn up 250 more (a half-hour of moderate jogging) than you usually do.

#2. "DIET" FOOD

"Fat burns in the flame of carbohydrate."
If there were a needlepoint sampler in the office of Canyon Ranch dietitian Linda Connell, that's what it would say. What it means is that in order to burn fat through exercise, you have to eat a diet high in carbohydrates, which are converted to glycogen, which provides energy. If your diet is too low in carbohydrates, you'll start to feel tired and maybe even lightheaded, but if you replenish your fuel supply—with an apple, for instance—you can keep going. The cycle is this: if you eat more carbohydrates, you can exercise more and use more fat. (In Chapter 13 there is much more about carbohydrates and the other food groups as well.)

#3. TIMING

Dietitians tell us that breakfast is the most important meal of the day, that we should never skip meals, and we should have our lightest meal at night. Since we're a nation of notorious breakfast-skippers who do some of our best eating while watching late-night TV, it's no wonder we're carrying around a lot of extra pounds.

Change your mealtime habits if you can, but if you can't, consider a compromise. Have a little something when you get up in the morning, then "graze" for the rest of the day—lots of small low-fat, high-carbohydrate meals. If you must eat at night, make it an apple or some other low-fat, high-carb food.

#4. PROFESSIONAL HELP

Just about everyone can use a little help when it comes to fighting a weight problem, and sometimes the best help of all comes from an expert: a dietitian. Following general dietary guidelines and prescribed regimens can be useful, but there's nothing quite like a tailor-made eating plan that makes nutritional sense and takes your specific tastes and your schedule into account.

A dietitian (look for the "R. D.," which means Registered Dietitian, next to the person's name) should examine your eating habits, recommend exercise as well as diet, and give you a diet that consists of a wide variety of foods that are low in fat, high in carbohydrates and fiber, and moderate in sodium, sugar, caffeine, and alcohol. A dietitian should not offer any diagnosis; sell supplements; make rash promises, such as fast and easy weight loss; or say she can cure you of an illness. The diet she gives you should be individualized, not preprinted, and unless a doctor has specifically instructed it, it should consist of no fewer than 1000 calories a day.

#5. TAKING IT SLOW

It's possible to lose ten pounds in two weeks, but you probably won't lose them for long. You're much better off losing ten pounds in ten weeks. True, losing weight slowly is a frustrating business, but if you want the weight to stay off, the slow and steady method is the only way to go. Safe weight loss occurs at an average of 1 percent of body weight per week; if you're at 170 now, losing 1.7 pounds a week is about right.

Keep in mind that weight loss is not always steady even if your willpower is. Some people who lose a lot of weight suddenly get stalled, often because their BMR is changing. The best thing to do is take a vacation from your diet for a while; stop trying to lose weight and concentrate on maintaining your new weight. After a month or two at the new weight you'll be ready for the last mile.

#6. BEHAVIOR MODIFICATION

Any standard weight-reduction technique will probably work over the short run, but the only one that works over time is changing your habits.

The only way to maintain a lower weight than your body is used to is not to let yourself return to a normal food pattern. The principle of behavior modification—instead of doing something undesirable and bad we should do something desirable and good—is so simple and so obvious, it's hard to believe that it was invented only about 15 years ago. Behavior modification has helped people deal with all sorts of bad habits, from drug dependency and phobias to procrastination and stress. In the area of weight control it involves modifying your thinking and your attitudes about food and exercise. (In Chapter 14 we explore the subject of behavior modification in depth.)

For most people this task is considerably easier said than done, and even if you win the battle, you still have to wage the war. One of the many Ranch staff members who knows something about the on-going struggle with weight is Ron Limoges, the director of the Canyon Ranch Foundation. Once a 300-pound compulsive eater who routinely ordered several room-service meals when he travelled on business and never got any exercise, Ron has lost more than 100 pounds and has given up his sedentary ways. It's been two years since he turned his life around, but he doesn't dare let down his guard when it comes to food, and he doesn't think he'll ever be able to. "I mostly eat the right things, but I'm still seriously addicted to food," he says. "I think about it all the time."

Like most people who have been on way too many diets, Ron knows that forever is a long time when it comes to weight loss. "There is one thing I'm sure of," he concludes philosophically. "When I die, I'm going to be either hungry or fat."

13

Four years and 65 pounds ago, Jack Stern, the first Canyon Ranch medical director, used to eat a pound bag of potato chips on the ten-minute drive home from work. Then he was ready for dinner, preferably a thick steak with all the trimmings. At 230 pounds, Jack was used to being fat; he remembered being the only kid in the seventh grade wearing a double-breasted suit. During college and medical school his weight continued to creep up, and later, as his practice grew, so did he. Then one day, as he tells it, Dr. Jack Stern got hit on the head with a two-by-four: he found out he had thyroid cancer.

Eighteen months later he had lost 65 pounds and lowered his cholesterol by 50 points, and he was exercising about two hours a day. He had also become an expert in nutrition. Fortunately for him, he had a secret weapon, a wife who was determined to learn all she could about the way to eat well. She took classes, read books and pamphlets, and began to explore the mysteries of the local health food store. She realized that it wasn't enough to make a commitment to eat well; you have to know exactly what that means.

Most of us *don't* know what that means. One of the things that is a constant source of surprise to the dietitians at the Ranch is how little people know about food and its effects on weight and overall health. When it comes to nutrition, we are a study in misinformation, just the way the Sterns were when they started out.

In the next few chapters we'll do what we can to set you straight about the best way to feed your body. In Chapter 14 we'll describe specific ways of evaluating and modifying your diet. Then in Chapter 15 we'll move on to managing your eating habits. But first let's talk about the nutritional basics.

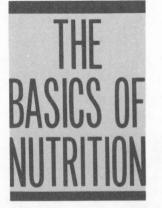

THE BASICS OF NUTRITION

According to the latest medical and nutritional research concerning preventive medicine and longevity, our diet should be high in complex carbohydrates and fiber and low in saturated fats, salt, and sugar. Caffeine and alcohol consumption should be moderate. The calorie breakdown that is generally recommended is 60 percent carbohydrates, 20 percent protein, and 20 percent fat. The standard American diet is more like 25 percent carbohydrates, 35 percent protein, and 40 percent fat, the fiber content is low, and we consume too much salt, sugar, caffeine, and alcohol. Let's take the elements one at a time.

CARBOHYDRATES

The rich get richer, and the poor get carbohydrates. That used to be the thinking, when people who couldn't afford meat had to live on spaghetti, potatoes, beans, grains, and bread. Of course, we didn't know then what we know now: that a bowl of spaghetti, a baked potato, a crusty roll, or a plate of rice and stir-fried vegetables are a lot better for us than the finest cut of prime meat. All the starchy "fattening" foods that Grandma thought she had to pass up are in fact the new heroes of nutrition. Now we know that you don't get fat from eating carbohydrates; you get fat from eating fat. Whether you want to gain weight, lose weight, or build muscle, carbohydrates should be the staple of your diet.

Before you start fantasizing about a diet that revolves around jelly doughnuts, keep in mind that there are two kinds of carbohydrates: *complex*, which are the starches; and *simple*, which are the sugars. As you probably have guessed, it is the complex carbohydrates that you should be eating—fruits, vegetables, grains, rice, beans, pasta, whole grain breads— not the sugary doughnuts and candy bars. Complex carbohydrates have a stabilizing effect on the system, since they are digested more slowly than simple carbohydrates; starchy foods have a healthy stick-to-the-ribs quality. Because simple carbohydrates are digested quickly, they have a pronounced, and undesirable, effect on the blood sugar. If you don't believe it, remember how you feel a half-hour after eating a candy bar.

Complex carbohydrates are the body's most readily used energy source; carbohydrates are converted to glycogen, which is used for energy. Carbs fuel the body so that we can breathe, move our muscles, keep ourselves warm, digest our food, repair bodily tissue, and maintain our immune system. Carbohydrates are also essential for burning fat and losing weight.

WHAT WE RECOMMEND

At the Ranch 60 percent of the calories we serve come from complex carbohydrates: fruits, vegetables, grains, and legumes. Except for a small amount of fructose we serve virtually no simple carbohydrates. Most people aren't that abstemious at home, but we do recommend that simple carbohydrates should make up no more than 15 percent of the total number of calories.

PROTEIN

Protein is the stuff of life. Roughly three-fourths of the body's tissue—muscles, organs, antibodies, enzymes, and some hormones—are composed of protein, and so is hemoglobin, which carries oxygen through the bloodstream. We need protein to build, maintain, and repair tissue, and it's also used as an energy source when carbohydrates and fats are not available.

Although protein is vital to the body's function, you don't really need very much of it. Most men eat too much protein; many women eat too little. The need for protein in both sexes is really quite modest: four to six ounces a day. However, because the excess can't be stored as protein, you can't eat half a chicken on Monday and let it take you through the week. Excess protein is stored as fat, not protein; you need to replenish protein stores every day.

Since muscles are made of protein, it stands to reason that if you want to build muscles, you should load up on protein, right? Wrong. Contrary to myth, protein does not build muscles; only exercise does that. Even if you're the most avid of bodybuilders, you still need only about six ounces of protein a day. The extra energy you may need to pump iron should come from complex carbohydrates.

Ounce for ounce meat, fish, poultry, seafood, and dairy products are the most "efficient" sources of protein—they're between 15 and 40 percent protein—but they're also the highest in fat. Cereals, beans, nuts, soybeans, and vegetables contain protein too, but only 3 to 10 percent. Obviously you have to eat more of the vegetable protein than the animal protein to fill your daily needs.

WHAT WE RECOMMEND

The recommended daily allowance of protein for adults is .8 grams of protein for each 2.2 pounds of body weight. At Canyon Ranch our menu is 20 percent protein, much of which comes from beans, legumes, grains, and vegetables as well as a little animal protein. We encourage our guests to use high-fat protein sources sparingly and explore the wonders of vegetable protein.

FATS

Fats, the primary fuel used during prolonged aerobic exercise, provide the most concentrated and abundant form of energy in the body. They also give us insulation, transport vitamins throughout the body, and keep our skin looking good. That's the good news. The bad news is that fat clogs the arteries, making it harder for blood to flow through the body. Fat also makes you fat. Some fats are better than others, however. Here's how they break down.

SATURATED FATS

Saturated fats—the animal fats plus coconut, palm, and palm kernel oil—are the true nutritional villains. As we've discussed in earlier chapters, eating saturated fats clogs your arteries, raises your overall cholesterol levels, and stimulates the production of LDL cholesterol. In fact, saturated fats elevate blood cholesterol more than dietary cholesterol itself; thus palm oil is worse for you than eggs or shellfish.

One way to remember which fats are saturated is to know that they're the ones that are solid at room temperature. The more solid a fat is, the more saturated it is; thus sticks are more saturated than tubs, which in turn are more saturated than liquids. The exceptions are the tropical oils, coconut, palm, and palm kernel, which are highly saturated yet liquid at room temperature.

UNSATURATED FATS

These are the "good fats," and here again there are two kinds: monounsaturated and polyunsaturated. Both kinds tend to lower blood cholesterol, but because monounsaturated fats (olive oil and peanut oil) lower LDL cholesterol without bringing down the HDL, they are generally considered to be better for you. Polyunsaturated fats, among them safflower, sunflower, corn, and canola oil, may lower HDL as well as LDL.

What's more, highly polyunsaturated fats are unstable; recent research indicates that when you heat these polyunsaturates, they liberate chemical substances called free radicals. Free radicals are produced naturally by the body, but too many can be dangerous, possibly carcinogenic. To be safe use monounsaturates for cooking and always store polyunsaturated fats in the refrigerator.

WHAT WE RECOMMEND

The fact is that in a well-balanced diet we get plenty of fat from our protein sources; we really don't need any extra fat. Certainly we don't need much of the foods that are mostly fat: mayonnaise, nuts and seeds, butter, margarine, sour cream, oil, olives, avocado, cream cheese, and salad dressings.

The American Cancer Society says that 30 percent of our calories should come from fat. The National Academy of Sciences says that 35 percent should be the limit. According to Nathan Pritikin, the magic number is 10. At the Ranch we say 20 percent is the number to shoot for, mostly because we know that a lower number just isn't realistic. We try to send our guests away with the determination to keep all fat low and to make olive and canola the oils of choice.

We know that a low-fat diet can literally undo the effects of a high-fat diet, so one of the most important dietary changes you can make is to lower your fat intake. We discuss many specific strategies for doing this in Chapter 14.

FIBER

One of the most important of all nutrients is, in fact, a *non*-nutrient, something the body can't even digest. It's fiber, and unless you've been living on another planet for the last few years, you've probably heard about it. Dietary fiber is the residue from plant cell walls (animal products do not contain fiber) that is not digestible in the small intestine. Touted as laxative, diet aid, skin toner, and all-around elixir, fiber is clearly the food whose time has come.

Even so, the average American diet is woefully short on fiber; most of us eat about 12 grams a day, and practically no one has more than 20 grams. There is no official USRDA (United States Recommended Daily Allowance) on fiber as yet, but the National Cancer Institute says that we should be eating 25 to 35 grams a day. Other experts say 30 to 50 grams is more like it.

There are two kinds of fiber, but fiber isn't as complicated as fats; both are good.

INSOLUBLE FIBER

This kind, the one that used to be called "roughage," is found in whole grains, wheat bran, beans, fruits, and vegetables. By absorbing water (which is why it's called insoluble) and increasing bulk, insoluble fiber relieves and prevents constipation, diverticulosis, appendicitis, hemorrhoids, obesity, irritable bowel syndrome, and cancer of the breast, prostate, and colon.

SOLUBLE FIBER

Soluble fiber (which dissolves in water) is relatively new on the nutritional scene. It has come into favor lately because of its newly discovered ability to lower blood cholesterol and its effectiveness in controlling adult onset diabetes. The best source of soluble fiber is oat bran and rolled oats, but it is also found in dried beans, unpeeled fruit, and raw vegetables. In addition to its cholesterol-lowering abilities it slows the absorption of carbohydrates and produces a more even rise in blood sugar after you eat. The feeling of fullness you are left with may make it easier to control your weight.

WHAT WE RECOMMEND

The Canyon Ranch menu is high in fiber, mostly from unrefined complex carbohydrates, especially oatmeal, brown rice, lentils, dried beans, bran, whole wheat flour, fruits, and vegetables. We encourage our guests to shoot for 25 to 35 grams a day, and we discourage the use of the new fiber pills on the market. They don't actually contain much fiber—no more than an apple or two—and they may interfere with the absorption of other nutrients.

. Chapter 14 has specific information about how to increase the fiber in your diet.

A WORD ABOUT WATER

At Canyon Ranch you don't have any trouble getting a glass of water with your meals. In fact, you get a full pitcher of it, complete with a server determined to fill your glass whenever the level drops even a little. Here in our desert oasis we take our water seriously; everywhere you look there is a pitcher of water or a water fountain or a trail leader offering you a canteen. We encourage our guests to drink at least 64 ounces of water a day, but we (and they) are happier if they drink much more. We hope they get into the habit of drinking water and keep it up when they get home.

Water cools the body, improves circulation and digestion, and fuels our muscles; we need water as much as we need air. Dehydration can be caused by a long list of things; alcohol, caffeine, sugar, smoking, sun, wind, heat, air conditioning, and exercise all conspire to rob the body of water. One of the biggest fitness favors you can do for yourself is to get into the habit of drinking several glasses of water every day.

SUGAR

On the one hand, sugar isn't quite so bad for us as we used to think. It doesn't cause heart disease or cancer or even diabetes, and it has only four calories a gram—the same as protein. On the other hand, it does cause tooth decay, and those four calories are virtually useless: no vitamins, no minerals, no fiber, no protein, just calories. What's more, where there is sugar, there is usually fat as well.

Sugar shows up in the most unlikely places: cereals, canned vegetables, fruit juices, soups, all sorts of processed foods. What's more, sugar travels under a lot of assumed names, but no matter what you call it, it's still sugar.

♦ Sucrose. This is the name given to table sugar, the kind we sprinkle on our cereal, and confectioner's sugar. It comes from sugar cane or sugar beets and contains 46 calories a tablespoon. Sucrose produces a fast and high rise in your blood sugar level, followed by an equally fast drop.

♦ Honey. Honey is made of fructose, glucose, maltose, and sucrose. Slightly less sweet than sucrose with a few trace nutrients, it has 65 calories a tablespoon.

♦ Brown sugar. This is sucrose colored with molasses; the darker it is, the more molasses it has. At 52 calories a tablespoon it is not as refined as table sugar, but it's about as nutritious.

♦ Fructose. This sugar, naturally found in fruit, is almost twice as sweet as sucrose, and it provides a less dramatic rise and fall of the blood sugar level than sucrose. Fructose contains 46 calories per tablespoon, the same as sucrose.

♦ Sorghum syrup. This is a mixture of sucrose, glucose, and fructose. It has 51 calories a tablespoon.

♦ Barley malt syrup. This sugar, a mix of maltose and glucose, contains 59 calories per tablespoon.

♦ Molasses. A combination of sucrose, fructose, and glucose, molasses has anywhere from 43 (for blackstrap) to 50 calories per tablespoon. It's drawn from sugar crystals as they are refined into pure sucrose.

WHAT WE RECOMMEND

If life were perfect, we would all give up sugar entirely, but life, as you probably know, isn't perfect. At the Ranch we use sugar very sparingly, and when we do add it to our recipes, we use fructose, for two reasons. First, since it's twice as sweet as table sugar, we can use less of it to sweeten food; and second, it's absorbed into the system more slowly than sucrose—causing a 20 percent rise in blood sugar, as opposed to the 60 percent rise you get with table sugar or honey.

We provide artificial sweeteners (and prefer aspartame) but we don't really like them because we can't be sure of what those chemicals do to the body. We're realistic enough to know that our guests can't go without the sweetness of sugar entirely but optimistic enough to encourage them to cut down. (There's more about lowering sugar consumption in Chapter 14.)

SODIUM

The verdict is not yet in on the evils of sodium, but there has been a lot of evidence presented, and much of it points to the fact that a diet high in sodium is associated with hypertension, which in turn is associated with heart attacks and strokes. The American Heart Association says that we should aim for no more than 3500 milligrams of sodium per day.

WHAT WE RECOMMEND

On the Canyon Ranch plan our guests consume between one and two grams of sodium a day. We encourage them to flavor their foods with seasonings other than salt. (For more about a low-salt diet, see Chapter 14.)

ALCOHOL

Alcohol is mostly simple carbohydrates, which we've already covered, but because of its far-reaching effects on health, we've put it in a category by itself. Chemically alcohol is ethyl alcohol, a depressant drug that slows the activity of the brain and spinal cord. It enters the bloodstream rapidly and circulates to all parts of the body within a few minutes. Metabolically speaking, alcohol can play havoc with your diet, because the calories that come from alcohol are metabolized before any others. Thus if you have a few drinks before dinner, those calories have to be used up before your body can even start on the entrée. Drinking adds pounds in other ways too, by increasing your appetite and decreasing your inhibitions, a dangerous combination when it comes to controlling weight.

Alcohol does a lot more than make you fat. It can aggravate osteoporosis, give you an upset stomach, dehydrate you, and make you anemic. It can cause diarrhea, give you low blood sugar, and act as a vasodilator (making your face blotchy or red). Alcohol also inhibits your body's ability to use certain nutrients, especially zinc, potassium, and magnesium, and alters the rate of absorption of calcium, folic acid, vitamins B6 and B12, and thiamine. It changes the metabolism of Vitamin D, causes liver fat to accumulate, blocks protein synthesis, and increases acid excretion in the stomach, which causes inflammation of the stomach lining.

Excessive use of alcohol can damage nearly every function and organ of your body, especially the heart. Heavy alcohol consumption damages healthy heart muscle, puts extra strain on an already damaged heart, and increases blood pressure. Current estimates are that alcohol intake accounts for 5 to 25 percent of all essential hypertension. (See Chapter 3.) Very heavy drinkers—those who have six or more drinks a day—who go on the wagon typically lower their blood pressure by more than ten points almost immediately. Cutting down on drinking usually leads to weight loss, which also has a positive effect on blood pressure.

WHAT WE RECOMMEND

At the Ranch we don't serve alcohol, and we strongly suggest that our guests have no more than a couple of drinks a day when they get home. (There's more about how to decrease your alcohol intake in Chapter 14.)

CAFFEINE

What's the most widely used drug in the United States? Here's a hint: it's also one of the most powerful, most addictive, and most sociably acceptable of all drugs. It's caffeine.

There is still much to learn about the effects of caffeine on the human body (the biggest question at the moment is whether or not it causes lumps in the breast), but so far the news is not great. A central nervous system stimulant, caffeine makes your heart pump faster and your breath come quicker, and it may increase your basal metabolic rate. Too much of it may cause calcium loss and make you jittery and restless. Other effects are insomnia, headaches, heart palpitations, and panic attacks. It does its job quickly, too; caffeine can move into your bloodstream in as little as 15 minutes and keep working for as long as two hours.

WHAT WE RECOMMEND

In most healthy people a moderate daily intake of caffeine—about 300 milligrams, which translates into two or three cups of coffee or five cups of strong tea—does no real harm. (We also get caffeine in cola, chocolate, and prescription and nonprescription drugs.) Still, at the Ranch we take the position that caffeine is not healthful. The coffee we serve is decaffeinated.

Most people who kick the caffeine habit suffer some withdrawal symptoms, usually off-and-on minor headaches for a few days. In other, relatively rare cases the withdrawal process is longer and much more difficult, involving digestive upsets, sleep disorders, and pains in the muscles and joints. Withdrawal from caffeine is by no means a totally physical matter. Like another stimulant, cigarette smoking, drinking coffee is a "relaxing" ritual, because you let yourself relax when you do it. That's why it's called a coffee break. (We talk more about how the physical and the psychological aspects of caffeine withdrawal in Chapter 14.)

VITAMINS AND MINERALS

Protein, carbohydrates, and fat make up the macronutrients; vitamins and minerals are the micronutrients. *Micro* doesn't mean that vitamins and minerals are any less important to good nutrition than the macronutrients; in fact, they are indispensable. Both vitamins and minerals are necessary for the metabolism of carbohydrates, proteins, and fats to produce energy. Calcium, magnesium, phosphorus, sulphur, sodium, potassium, and chlorine are necessary in bulk; we need trace elements of iron, zinc, copper, manganese, chromium, iodine, selenium, molybdenum, and cobalt; and ultratrace amounts of vanadium, rubidium, lithium, arsenic, nickel, and lead are necessary.

Here are the recommended daily allowances of the most significant vitamins and minerals:

NUTRIENT	USRDA
VITAMIN A	5000 IU (International Units)
VITAMIN B1 (THIAMINE)	1.5 mg. (milligrams)
VITAMIN B6	2 mg.
VITAMIN B12	4 mcg. (micrograms)
VITAMIN C	60 mg.
VITAMIN D	400 IU
VITAMIN E	30 IU
CALCIUM	1000 mg.
IRON	18 mg.
MAGNESIUM	400 mg.
ZINC	15 mg.
POTASSIUM	1800–5000 mg.
VITAMIN B2 (RIBOFLAVIN)	1.7 mg.
VITAMIN B3 (NIACIN)	20 mg.
FOLIC ACID	400 mcg.
VITAMIN B5 (PANTOTHENIC ACID)	10 mg.
CHROMIUM	No RDA; 50–200 mcg.
COPPER	2 mg.
SELENIUM	No RDA; 50–200 mcg.

Naturally, each vitamin and mineral fills a specific function in the well-balanced diet: the B vitamins help the nervous system, Vitamin E is good for the skin, iron is vital for oxygen transport, sodium and potassium help maintain your water balance, and so on. One important mineral that has been in the spotlight lately is calcium.

CALCIUM

Calcium is so important, our bodies will actually rob our bones to get it if necessary. Calcium is vital for strong bones and teeth, muscle contraction, blood clotting, transmission of nerve impulses, regulation of the heart rhythms, and the chemical activity of all the body's cells. An adequate calcium intake also helps prevent osteoporosis, a loss of bone mass associated with aging, which plagues more than half the women in this country over the age of 65.

It's no wonder that calcium has become downright fashionable, with everything from soft drinks to fast-food hamburger buns claiming to be fortified with the miracle mineral. Total sales of calcium supplements are more than $160 million a year; the year the word got out that Tums, which had previously been known only as an antacid tablet, was a good source of calcium, sales increased by 40 percent.

Men and premenopausal women need about 1000 milligrams a day of calcium; women past menopause need more, about 1200 to 1500 milligrams. In general we don't get nearly enough; the average woman consumes about 550 milligrams of calcium a day.

There are several effective ways to increase your daily intake of calcium:

♦ Food. The best source of calcium is food, specifically dairy products and preferably low-fat ones, such as skim milk, low-fat yogurt, and low-fat cheese. Non-dairy sources of calcium are salmon, sardines (with the bones), oysters, shrimp, soybeans, rutabagas, broccoli, oranges, tofu, and kale, collard, turnip, and mustard greens.

♦ Exercise. Exercise doesn't actually introduce calcium into the body, but it does increase the body's ability to absorb calcium. Weight-bearing activity, such as walking and running, is almost as good for the bones as a glass of milk.

♦ Calcium supplements. Some people, especially women, just can't get enough calcium through their diets. If you're one of them, you might want to consider taking a calcium supplement, provided your doctor approves. (Calcium pills may cause kidney stones. They may also lower your blood pressure and interfere with the actions of other medication.) There are dozens of supplements on the market these days, so look closely at what you're getting. Calcium carbonate and calcium citrate are the cheapest, and they also contain the most calcium. Avoid fortified supplements and stay away from added bone meal and dolomite. Don't take more than 1000 milligrams of elemental calcium a day; a dose of 500 is probably plenty, and it's best spread out over the day—250 in the morning and 250 at night.

VITAMIN AND MINERAL SUPPLEMENTS

Wouldn't it be great if we could just take a pill and be healthy? That's exactly what the manufacturers of vitamin and mineral supplements would like you to think you can do. To hear them tell it, extra vitamins will make you stronger, sexier, healthier, and even smarter and they'll cure everything from baldness to stress. The truth is that the only people who need vitamin or mineral supplements are women who are pregnant or breast-feeding, strict vegetarians, people on unbalanced or very low-calorie diets, or people whose physicians say they should. If you eat a well-balanced diet of 1600 to 2000 calories a day, you are probably getting all the nutrients you need from your food.

Having said that, we should also say that taking a daily multivitamin-mineral tablet is not likely to do you any harm, especially if your diet is erratic or you're counting calories. (Many women don't get enough iron in their diets.) However, if you start playing around with individual vitamin and mineral supplements, you run the risk of upsetting your nutritional balance. For instance, too much copper may interfere with the absorption of zinc; too much Vitamin C may interfere with the absorption of copper; and large doses of Vitamin C in women may reduce fertility. Megadoses of some vitamins, especially Vitamins A and D, may be toxic.

WHAT WE RECOMMEND

The suggested menu at the Ranch gives our guests a well-balanced diet, but because people may choose instead to create their own menus (see Chapter 24) and add or subtract calories, we offer two multi-vitamin and mineral tablets each morning. These two tablets provide 100 to 250 percent of the USRDA for most adults.

DIET AND CANCER

We've come a long way in our knowledge of nutrition; we know a great deal about how what we eat affects our health. But we still have a lot to learn, especially about diet and cancer prevention. Researchers' progress has been slow, and much of what we know has come indirectly, from studies of how various populations eat and what effect their diet appears to have on their health. (For instance, in Japan, where women eat only 15 to 20 percent of their calories as fat, the incidence of breast cancer is quite low.) We've gotten the rest of our data from test tube experiments and studies of how various foods affect laboratory animals. Since humans are neither lab animals nor test tubes, the results of many of the studies are inconclusive, to say the least.

Still, experts have concluded, however tentatively, that some foods may prevent cancer and others may increase your chances of developing it. In 1984 the American Cancer Society went so far as to issue guidelines for a cancer-preventive diet, which said that in general we should be eating more fruits, vegetables, and grains and less fat, cholesterol, sugar, and sodium. The guidelines also contained some specific suggestions about the heroes and villains in the nutritional world.

THE GOOD GUYS

The following foods may offer some protection against cancer:

♦ Fiber. Fruits, vegetables, legumes, and whole grains are particularly helpful in promoting healthy bowel function.

♦ Cruciferous vegetables. We should be eating two or three servings per week of the members of the cabbage family, such as broccoli, kale, brussels sprouts, and cauliflower.

♦ Beta carotene. Eventually transformed into Vitamin A, beta carotene is found in yellow, orange, and green leafy vegetables and fruit, especially carrots, cantaloupe, broccoli, yams, and spinach.

♦ Vitamin A. We need about 5000 international units of Vitamin A every day. Vitamin A is available naturally in liver, butter, milk, cheese, egg yolks, and fish oil. Megadoses of Vitamin A can be toxic, so you should avoid supplements.

♦ Vitamin C. We need about 60 milligrams of Vitamin C a day, the amount found in about four ounces of fresh juice. Again, megadoses can be dangerous, sometimes causing diarrhea or kidney stones. Good sources of Vitamin C are citrus fruits, tomatoes, broccoli, strawberries, potatoes, peppers, and kale.

♦ Vitamin E. This nutrient is available in nuts, vegetable oils, liver, margarine, whole grains, wheat germ, and dried beans. You get all the Vitamin E you need in one tablespoon of margarine.

♦ Selenium. Seafood, liver, meats, grains, egg yolks, and tomatoes contain selenium.

There is evidence that eating the following foods increases your chances of developing cancer:

♦ Fats. A diet too heavy in fat appears to cause cancer of the digestive and reproductive system. It also contributes to obesity, which is another risk factor for cancer.

♦ Alcohol. Heavy drinking—more than two drinks a day—may cause cancer of the mouth, throat, liver, bladder, and possibly the breast.

♦ Nitrites. The chemical used to preserve cured meats, such as bacon, hot dogs, sausages, and ham, has been shown to cause cancer in laboratory animals. You should limit your intake of those foods.

♦ Aflatoxins. If you see mold on peanuts, peanut butter, seeds, or corn, throw it out immediately. The mold appears to be carcinogenic.

♦ Charred foods. When meat is grilled, barbecued, or fried at high temperatures, cancer-causing agents are created. Steam, bake, roast, or cook your meat or fish in a microwave oven whenever possible.

Taking the Next Step

Unless you're planning to go on a game show some time soon, all of this nutritional information is useful only if you learn to put it to practical use, by taking a look at how you're eating now and learning how to accentuate the positive and eliminate the negative. That's what we'll explore in the next chapter.

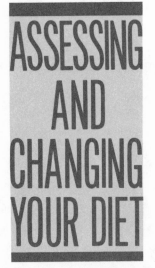

ASSESSING AND CHANGING YOUR DIET

Consider this: a typical serving of lasagna has about 650 calories. If you cut your portion in half, you'll save 325 calories. If you eat lasagna 25 times a year, that comes to an annual savings of 8125 calories, or 2.32 pounds a year.

Or this: nearly every Sunday morning you treat yourself to a big breakfast at your favorite diner. You usually have a glass of orange juice (120 calories), a cheese omelet (450) with hash browns (490), and toast with butter and jam (250). Breakfast comes to about 1200 calories. If you went to the same diner and ordered a bowl of fresh fruit and a stack of pancakes with syrup (sorry, no butter), your breakfast would come to about 800 calories, a 400-calorie saving. If you did this just 40 Sunday mornings a year, you'd cut 16000 calories from your diet and lose 4.57 pounds.

And this: if you did just those two things, changed your Sunday breakfast and cut your twice-monthly lasagna in half, you would lose 6.89 pounds a year, all without "dieting" or additional exercise.

In this chapter we're going to examine many such changes you can make in your diet, all designed to help you increase your intake of starch and fiber, cut down on your fat, sugar, and salt, and reduce your consumption of caffeine and alcohol. Some modifications will be easier than others, but they are all realistic. You probably won't be able to change all of your habits, and certainly not all at once, but if you take things one step at a time, you can make a big difference in your nutritional picture. The first step is to take a critical look at the way you eat now.

Taking a Look at Your Diet

The first thing the dietitians ask the Canyon Ranch guests is to describe a typical day of eating, and over the years, we've heard it all. Some people starve themselves all day, living on coffee and artificial sweetener, then eat nonstop all night. Many have a danish for breakfast, a salad for lunch, a candy bar in the afternoon, and a big dinner. Almost everyone has a healthier diet during the week than on the weekends. And then there was the man who was literally eating for two; his diet was quite well balanced, but he ate twice as much of everything as he needed.

During these nutritional assessments our guests learn as much as we do. Many of them realize that they're completely out of touch with what and how much they've been eating. In many instances they discover that they've been kidding themselves.

When Linda Connell, the head of the nutrition department, asked one man about his typical dinner, he said that he often had steak—"medium-sized," he explained. When Linda brought out her handy set of food models and asked him to show her the size of his steak, the story became quite different. His "medium-sized" steak was, in fact, mammoth; it came to about 1600 calories, two thirds of the total he needed for the day. For fewer than half those calories he could have been eating six ounces of broiled fish, a baked potato, a serving of broccoli, and a salad with Italian dressing.

Even people with the best intentions can make nutritional mistakes. One woman's daily breakfast consisted of orange juice and a cup of fruit-and-nut granola with milk and a sliced banana—quite nutritious, she thought. If she switched to an orange and a cup of shredded wheat with skim milk and that same sliced banana, she would be getting more fiber, a lot less fat and cholesterol, and 211 fewer calories.

Another well-meaning woman said she always has a chef's salad when she goes out to lunch, little knowing that those strips of ham, cheese, turkey, and roast beef, not to mention the dressing and the other trimmings, comes to about 1200 calories. If she orders a turkey sandwich with mustard and lettuce, she'll save more than 700 calories a day. (She could have two turkey sandwiches and still be 200 calories better off.)

Before you can begin to reform your eating habits, you should know where your calories come from. If you don't realize that there are 490 calories in that cup of hash browns—a serving some people can gobble down without even noticing—you could be sabotaging your efforts. Look at what you're eating. A baked potato contains about 200 high-fiber, low-fat calories, but by the time you add a tablespoon of butter and a couple of tablespoons of sour cream to the potato, you're up to 400 calories.

Eating eight ounces of potato chips is like adding 15 teaspoons of hydrogenated vegetable oil and a teaspoon of salt to a baked potato.

For the same number of calories in three ounces of cheddar cheese you can eat six oranges, five slices of bread, or fifteen cups of broccoli. Of course, if it's cheese you really want, even a hundred cups of broccoli won't satisfy you. There are times when we cry out for specific types of food, and nothing else will do.

UNDERSTANDING YOUR HUNGERS

Salad dressing makes salad wet and adds flavor. So does lemon juice or vinegar or diluted blue cheese dressing. Tuna fish salad cries out for a substance to hold it together and make it spreadable, something low-fat yogurt can do just as well as all-fat mayo. Look at the function of that topping on your baked potato. If you add butter and sour cream to make it wet and flavorful, maybe you would be just as happy with stewed tomatoes or mustard instead.

If you're going to make dietary changes you can live with, you can't just take things out of your diet; a plain baked potato or a naked salad just won't do for most people. You have to put things in as well. Here are some substitutes for our most popular taste and texture sensations:

♦ Creamy smooth. Instead of ice cream or pudding, try applesauce, mashed squash, a soft-boiled egg, oatmeal, low-fat yogurt, or a ripe banana.

♦ Chewy. Try dates, raisins, and other dried fruit, bagels, or taffy. A day-old pumpernickel bagel has more chew per ounce than almost any other food.

♦ Crunchy. Instead of corn chips choose breadsticks, popcorn, pretzels, rice cakes, radishes, pretzel sticks, or celery.

♦ Sour. Choose pickles or cucumbers in vinegar.

♦ Sweet. All fruits are sweet, but the sweetest are grapes, cherries, bananas, and ripe peaches. Oatmeal sweetened with apple butter and frozen yogurt are also satisfying.

Now let's move into the specific ways of changing your diet for the better.

#1. REDUCE FAT

Fat is everywhere, in your meat, your cookies, your muffins, the sauce on your vegetables, even in that "diet platter" you thought you ordered.

Bacon and baloney are 83 percent fat; hot dogs are 75 percent fat; ice cream is 61 percent fat; chocolate chip cookies are about half fat. That fish you had for dinner may have been low in fat (salmon is 54 percent fat, but sole is 6 percent), but the sauce probably wasn't. That handful and a half of peanuts you ate without even realizing it had more than 500 calories, 75 percent of which come from fat.

We're not trying to depress you with all of these numbers; we're just trying to open your eyes with a few sobering facts. When it comes to the fat in food, there are plenty more facts where they came from.

RATING THE OILS

All fats and oils are created equal when it comes to calories—nine per gram, to be exact—but as we explained in Chapter 13, unsaturated fats are considerably better for you than saturated fats. Here's how the most commonly used fats and oils rate.

OIL OR FAT	% SATURATED	% UNSATURATED MONO-	POLY-
CANOLA	8	57	35
SAFFLOWER	9	13	78
SUNFLOWER	11	21	68
CORN	13	25	62
SOYBEAN	15	25	60
SESAME	14	42	44
PEANUT	18	48	34
OLIVE	14	77	9
COTTONSEED	27	18	55
MARGARINE	19	53	28
SHORTENING	25	68	7
LARD	41	43	16
BUTTER	68	28	4
PALM	53	38	9
COCONUT	92	6	2

DAIRY PRODUCTS

Getting enough calcium in your diet can be a high-calorie and high-fat business if you're not careful. A cup of skim milk, an ounce and a half of cheese, a cup and three quarters of ice cream, two cups of 2 percent cottage cheese, one cup of plain low-fat yogurt, and a cup of pudding all contain roughly the same amount of calcium, but the calorie counts are miles apart: skim milk, 80 calories; cheese, 174; ice cream, 610; cottage cheese, 406; yogurt, 125; and pudding, 340.

SO WHAT SHOULD YOU PUT ON YOUR TOAST?

BUTTER. One tablespoon of butter has 100 calories, 11 grams of fat, 7 grams saturated fat, and (because it's animal fat) 35 milligrams of cholesterol.

MARGARINE. Margarine is a vegetable fat that has been hydrogenated to make it solid enough to spread. (The more solid it is—in stick as opposed to tub form—the more saturated fat it contains.) A tablespoon of margarine has about 100 calories, 11 grams of fat, 2 grams of saturated fat, and (because it's not animal fat) no cholesterol.

MARGARINE/BUTTER BLENDS. These are just what they sound like. A tablespoon has 90 calories, 10 grams of fat, 4 grams of saturated fat, and about 5 milligrams of cholesterol.

VEGETABLE OIL SPREADS. The two best known brands are Promise and I Can't Believe It's Not Butter. A tablespoon has from 60 to 90 calories, 6 to 10 grams of fat, 1 or 2 grams of saturated fat, and no cholesterol.

DIET MARGARINE. A tablespoon of Weight Watchers diet margarine has 50 calories, 5 grams of fat, 1 gram of saturated fat, and no cholesterol.

JAMES AND JELLIES. If you're worried about fat consumption, your best bet is stop buttering your bread. A teaspoon of grape jelly or orange marmalade contains only about 17 calories, none of which come from fat.

Here are a few more interesting numbers. A cup of whole milk (about 160 calories) contains the fat equivalent of two pats of butter; 2 percent milk (120 calories a cup) has one pat removed; with 1 percent milk you're down to half a pat and about 100 calories; and skim milk, at 80 calories a cup, has all the butter removed.

Cheese is incredibly high in fat, especially Roquefort, swiss, Brie, monterey jack, and American cheese—all the ones we really love. However, there are a few relatively low-fat cheeses, with three grams of fat or less per ounce. If you have a craving for cheese, try low-fat cheddar, part-skim mozzarella, neufchatel (instead of cream cheese), part-skim ricotta, and low-fat cottage cheese.

LOW-FAT MEAT

Like cheese, meat is generally high in fat, and we encourage you to rely more on fish and chicken and less on red meat for your protein source. Still, there is nothing wrong with eating meat once in a while, as long as the portions are reasonable (no more than six ounces and preferably four), the cooking method is nutritionally sound (baked, roasted, or broiled, not fried), and the meat itself is relatively lean.

Spareribs and processed meats are about 80 percent fat, and many cuts of red meat are as high as 50 percent. However, there are a few caloric bargains in the butcher shop. Here's a list of some of the lower-fat cuts of meat.

"LIGHT" MEATS	% CALORIES FROM FAT	TOTAL CALORIES
Beef (4 OUNCES)		
CHUCK ARM OR ROUND-BONE, GRADED "GOOD," BRAISED	26	203
SIRLOIN, WEDGE OR ROUND-BONE, "GOOD," BROILED	26	208
ROUND STEAK, BROILED	29	215
SIRLOIN, DOUBLE-BONE, "GOOD," BROILED	29	216
PORTERHOUSE, "GOOD," BROILED	32	224
Lamb (4 OUNCES)		
FORESHANK, BRAISED	30	203
SHANK HALF OF LEG, ROASTED	34	199
Pork (4 OUNCES)		
LOIN, TENDERLOIN, ROASTED	26	189
Veal (4 OUNCES)		
ARM STEAK, BRAISED	21	215
CUTLET, FRIED	22	206
BLADE STEAK, BRAISED	25	208
SIRLOIN CHOP, BRAISED	26	222
RIB ROAST, ROASTED	32	181
LOIN CHOP, BRAISED	33	239

#2. INCREASE STARCH

If dietitians ever decide to build a statue to a food, they would definitely choose the complex carbohydrate. Complex carbohydrates, or starches, as we are used to thinking of them, are low in fat and sodium, high in fiber, and satisfying to the appetite. In many countries entire diets are built around rice, bread, potatoes, and vegetables, with a modest amount of protein and fat for flavor.

The starches we're most accustomed to eating are rice, potatoes, breads, and fruits and vegetables, but we would do well to expand our repertoire to include pasta, grains, beans, and legumes.

One cup of cooked pasta contains 200 calories, no cholesterol, little sodium, and less than a gram of fat, and it gives you about 10 percent of the USRDA for protein. Spinach pasta throws in a little Vitamin A as well, and whole wheat pasta contains more fiber, protein, and iron. In fact, if it weren't for the cream sauce and the cheese that we often put on our noodles, pasta would be just about perfect.

Dried pasta is as nutritious as fresh, and serving it more *al dente* than mushy means that the vitamins are more likely to be in the noodles than in the cooking water. For best results choose fruit, tomato, vegetable, or fish sauces instead of cream or meat toppings and go easy on the cheese, butter, and oil.

Grains—barley, brown rice, buckwheat groats, bulghur wheat, corn grits, millet, rye, and triticale, to name a few—are new to most people. At about 200 low-fat calories per cup, they are rich in carbohydrate and fiber and high in calcium and iron. They can be used as meat substitutes in soups and casseroles, and they make nutritious, filling side dishes.

#3. INCREASE FIBER

As we discussed in Chapter 13, fiber is wonderful for our health, but it's important to increase your daily fiber intake gradually, over a period of a few weeks. A sudden increase in fiber consumption can give the digestive system something of a shock, sometimes causing gas, bloating, constipation, or diarrhea. Drinking a great deal of water can help; the water helps the fiber expand in the digestive tract so that it can more easily move through the system.

Here are several ways you can quite easily increase your fiber intake:

♦ Think brown instead of white: whole-wheat flour instead of white flour, brown rice instead of white, and whole-grain pasta instead of white. If the taste of whole-wheat products is strange to you, consider compromising. Mix white rice or pasta with the whole-wheat version. When a recipe calls for flour, use half white and half whole-wheat flour. Buy whole-grain breads, crackers, and cereals and corn instead of flour tortillas.

♦ Eat fresh fruits, complete with edible skin and membranes, instead of canned.

♦ Choose fresh vegetables, preferably several different ones a day, and eat them raw or slightly steamed; overcooking robs vegetables of nutrients. Eat the skins and edible stalks.

♦ Substitute legumes and grains for meat. Serve bean and vegetable soups as a main course and add oat bran or wheat bran to casseroles and barley to soups.

♦ Eat fiber cereals for breakfast.

♦ Eat high-fiber snacks, such as popcorn and dried fruit.

#4. Eat Less Cholesterol

As we have already discussed, the best way to reduce your blood cholesterol level is to reduce saturated fats (see above), but if your cholesterol is high, you should monitor your consumption of dietary cholesterol as well. Limit your intake of all animal products, especially meat, egg yolks, shellfish, and organ meats. Use soft margarine and liquid vegetable oils instead of butter. (For more about how to lower cholesterol through diet turn to Chapter 3.)

#5. Cut Down on Sugar

Americans have a real love affair with sugar. At last count each of us was eating about 120 pounds of the stuff a year, something between 20 and 25 percent of our total calories. Much of the time we aren't even aware we're eating something sweet. Who could guess that a tablespoon of ketchup has a teaspoon of sugar?

Even when we know we're eating something sweet, we may be deceiving ourselves. A cup of sugar is 700 calories, and a cup of fat is 1600 calories, yet how many times when you had a craving for something sweet have you chosen something fat instead? When your sweet tooth kicks in and won't be denied, don't choose ice cream, cakes, cookies, and pies; it's true that they're sweet, but they're mostly fat. You're much better off going for something high in sugar: jelly beans, hard candies, licorice, and gum drops, for instance.

But this is supposed to be about cutting *down* on sugar, not indulging in it. Here are a few suggestions:

♦ Doctor your recipes. You can almost always cut the specified amount of sugar in half without hurting the recipe. Try using fruit juices, fruit concentrates, and fruit purées to sweeten your food. Buy a cookbook for diabetics and do some experimenting.

♦ Substitute fructose for table sugar.

♦ Wean yourself away from soft drinks and alcohol. Drink water, seltzer, and diluted fruit juice instead.

♦ If you must serve canned fruits, pick ones canned in water or juice rather than heavy syrup.

♦ Don't believe everything you read. When a recipe says "sugar-free" or "sugarless," that just means that no table sugar, or sucrose, has been added to the contents. As we said in Chapter 12, there are many other sugars besides sucrose, any of which can be in that container marked "sugar-free."

ARTIFICIAL SWEETENERS

Let's face the grim facts: if artificial sweeteners made us thin, ours would not be the fattest nation in the world. According to an American Cancer Society study, which involved more than 78000 women aged 50 to 69, long-term users of artificial sweeteners were more likely to *gain* weight than non-users over the course of a year.

There are several problems with artificial sweeteners: first, they don't satisfy hunger or make you feel full the way sugar does; second, they may in fact stimulate the appetite; and third, they are usually just added to a diet, not used to replace high-fat foods. How many times have you had artificially sweetened coffee with your slice of cake? While you're cutting down on sugar, you would do well to break the artificial sweetener habit too.

#6. REDUCE YOUR SALT INTAKE

The salt habit is one of the very few that's easy to break. True, it may not seem easy at first—when you think your food tastes a little funny—but the biological fact is that in a fairly short time you'll actually lose your taste for food that is very salty. People who have been on low-sodium diets for even a couple of months find that the salty foods they used to enjoy now taste downright unpleasant.

So keeping in mind that it only hurts for a little while, try these methods of cutting down on salt:

♦ Modify your recipes. Virtually no recipe is harmed by cutting the amount of salt recommended in half, especially if you use herbs and spices instead. Some particularly tasty non-salt flavor enhancers are lemon juice, pepper, garlic, onion, marjoram, rosemary, dry mustard, basil, thyme, oregano, caraway, and sesame seeds. For best results use a mortar and pestle to crush dried herbs and release their full flavor.

♦ Limit your intake of processed and packaged foods, especially canned soups and vegetables, noodle or rice mixes, luncheon meats, and TV dinners. If you must use canned vegetables, rinse them in water first to get rid of some of the salt.

♦ Avoid food prepared in brine, such as pickles, sauerkraut, and olives.

♦ Look out for salt in disguise. Like sugar, salt comes in many forms and under many names besides sodium chloride. Be on the lookout for

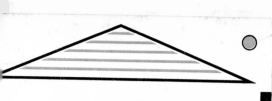

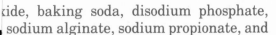

...xide, baking soda, disodium phosphate,
...sodium alginate, sodium propionate, and

...ubstitutes. Substitutes for salt, usually
...ve (about 17 dollars a pound, as opposed to
...eople they harm the kidneys and raise the

#7. CUT DOWN ON YOUR DRINKING

...ds this year without going on a diet, try
...ccording to the Department of Health and
...person over 14 years old in the United
...ee calories a year in wine, beer, and hard
...t. Here are some effective ways to cut that

...k. A moderate daily amount of alcohol is 3
...ries), 8 ounces of wine (220), or 24 ounces
...k at the drinks you've been pouring; the
...tankards have a lot to answer for.
...re than 5 ounces of wine, 12 ounces of beer,
... hour. If the drink is gone before the hour
...ave a glass of water. To make a drink last,
...ss down between sips.
...hen you have something to eat, the alcohol
...ore slowly, which means your judgment is
...lso means that you'll get some nutrients,
...eds when you're drinking.
...l occasions and times of great stress. When
...ense, you can lose track of how much you've

...olic, and preferably low in calories and fat,
...al cocktail. Diluted fruit juice can be very
... are the Canyon Ranch Mocktail (a glass of
sparkling water with a squeeze of fresh lemon or lime and a dash of
bitters, served with a lemon or lime wedge) and the Canyon Ranch
Margarita (blend until frothy a half-cup of crushed ice, eight ounces of
sparkling water, two tablespoons fresh lime juice, one tablespoon fructose,
and one egg white and serve over ice with a lime slice).

#8. CUT DOWN ON CAFFEINE

In the previous chapter we explained that 300 milligrams of caffeine is about as much as anyone should consume each day. Since a five-ounce cup of drip coffee has about 115 milligrams of caffeine (as opposed to tea, which has 60, and cocoa, which has 4), that probably means you should be cutting down on your coffee drinking. Here are some acceptable coffee substitutes.

♦ "Light coffee." Some people find that grain beverages, such as Postum, take the place of a morning cup of coffee quite nicely. Usually composed of bran, wheat, and molasses, they are low in calories and contain no caffeine. Others prefer to blend chicory or wheat with regular coffee; this is higher in caffeine than Postum but considerably lower than pure coffee.

♦ Herbal teas. At the Ranch we serve hundreds, sometimes thousands, of cups of herbal tea every day; some like it hot, and some like it cold. The favorites are Red Zinger, Mandarin Orange Spice, and Cinnamon Apple. As you make your choice, keep in mind that not all herbal teas are caffeine-free. For guests who must have a little caffeine in the morning we serve Morning Thunder, but there are other caffeinated herbal teas. Check the label before you buy. To sweeten iced herbal tea try an ounce or two of apple juice.

♦ Soft drinks. Colas and some citrus-flavored sodas contain caffeine (a 12-ounce can of cola has about 55 milligrams), but root beer, ginger ale, tonic water, and club soda do not.

♦ Decaffeinated coffee. This is something of a misnomer, since even decaf has a little caffeine, about four milligrams in a six-ounce cup, but all in all, decaf coffee is a pretty good alternative to the real thing. We serve water-washed decaffeinated coffee at the Ranch because we like the taste and don't like chemicals, but studies show that some chemically decaffeinated coffees are just fine too. If you're having trouble getting used to decaf, try a half-coffee, half-decaf blend.

#9. PLAN YOUR SNACKS

In the old days we weren't supposed to eat between meals, but today the thinking is that eating several small meals throughout the day—what we used to call between-meal snacks—may be the solution to our diet problems. Many people find that having an apple before leaving the office to go home or an hour before going to bed keeps them from overeating at other times. Naturally, some snacks are better than others. Here are some of the best.

CARBOHYDRATE SNACKS

SNACK	CARBOHYDRATES (gm)	CALORIES
1 ENGLISH MUFFIN*	41	183
1 CORN MUFFIN*	37	167
3 WASA CRISP BREAD	36	191
1 BRAN MUFFIN*	32	180
5 AK-MAK	30	125
4 LAHVOSH	30	140
4 RICE CAKES	30	140
1 BAGEL	30	160
14 3-RING PRETZELS	28	154
3 RYKRISP	27	90
5 RICE CRACKERS	27	100
4 BREAD STICKS	27	164
8 MELBA TOAST	26	122
2½ CUPS PLAIN POPCORN	26	115
5 GRAHAM CRACKERS	26	117
5 ZWEIBACK	26	156

FRUIT SNACKS

1 LARGE BANANA	40	160
1 MEDIUM ORANGE	20	80
1 LARGE APPLE	30	120
1 MEDIUM PEAR	30	120
4 MEDIUM DATES	30	115
7 APRICOT HALVES	27	106
2 FIGS	27	108
2 OUNCES RAISINS	28	104

SWEET SNACKS

15 JELLY BEANS	25	99
1 OUNCE GUMDROPS	25	99
2 ORANGE SLICES	31	125
13 ANIMAL CRACKERS	26	153
5 VANILLA WAFERS	14	85
2 FIG BARS	22	106
1 CREAMSICLE	18	103

* with 1 tablespoon jelly

LOW-CAL TOPPINGS It's all very well to tell you to fill up on rice cakes or snack on oatmeal and plain low-fat yogurt, but the reality is that most of us just don't like our cereals, crackers, bread, and other foods plain. Here are some low-fat toppings that will add some interest to your snacks.

TOPPING	CALORIES
1 TEASPOON VANILLA OR ALMOND EXTRACT	7
1 TABLESPOON APPLE OR GUAVA BUTTER	37
1 TABLESPOON MAPLE SYRUP	20
1 TABLESPOON APPLE CHUTNEY	41
1 TABLESPOON MUSTARD	11
1 TABLESPOON SWEET RELISH	21
1 TABLESPOON PART-SKIM PARMESAN CHEESE	33
2 TABLESPOONS LOW-FAT YOGURT	20

#10. LEARN TO READ FOOD LABELS

Sometimes you can't win for losing. The "natural" food you just brought home is artificial, "low-salt" foods may contain tons of sodium, many foods that are labeled "cholesterol-free" actually increase cholesterol, some all-beef hot dogs are just as fat-filled as their pork counterparts, and you just found out that the "naturally sweet" raisin bran you had for breakfast is almost half sugar. What's a health-conscious shopper to do?

Well, the first thing you have to do is not believe everything you read. The people who write food labels care less about your health than they do about selling their products. Ambiguous and misleading are the nicest things we can think of to say about most labels on packaged foods. Still, if you are going to take responsibility for your health, you have to learn to speak labelese. The following should get you started.

CALORIES

♦ Serving size. One of the ways food manufacturers make their products seem low in calories and fat is to fudge a little on the serving size. Before you decide that you've discovered a new diet food, look closely at the fine print and see how many people it's supposed to serve.

♦ "Low-calorie." Fewer than 40 calories per serving and fewer than .4 calories per gram.

♦ "Reduced-calorie." One third fewer calories than the regular version.

♦ "Diet" or "Dietetic." This means the same as either "low-calorie" or "reduced-calorie." They must contain no more than 40 calories per serving or have at least one third fewer calories than the regular product.

♦ "Light" (or "Lite"). No matter how it's spelled, it means absolutely nothing except when it describes processed meats. Then it means that the meat has 25 percent less fat than the usual model.

CHOLESTEROL

Remember, only animal products contain cholesterol, so a "no choles- terol" label can quite accurately be slapped on the side of any vegetable product. Remember too that no cholesterol does *not* mean no saturated fat, and saturated fat increases cholesterol more even than dietary cholesterol does. For example, peanut butter, margarine, and packaged coffeecakes made with hydrogenated vegetable oil (palm and coconut) have no cholesterol, but they're almost all fat.

♦ "Cholesterol-free." Fewer than 2 milligrams of cholesterol per serv- ing.

♦ "Low-cholesterol." Fewer than 20 milligrams of cholesterol per serving.

♦ "Cholesterol-reduced." The product has been reformulated so that it has 75 percent less cholesterol than the original.

♦ "Lower cholesterol." The cholesterol has been reduced but not by as much as 75 percent.

FAT

One of these days food manufacturers are going to be forced to spell out not just how much fat is in their products but also how much of it is saturated fat. Until that day comes, however, you have to read between the lines of the food labels. Look out for coconut, palm, and palm kernel oil and beware of the word "hydrogenated," which means that the fat is anything from 5 to 60 percent saturated. "Made with 100 percent vegetable shortening" could mean that there's canola or sesame oil in there, but it's much more likely to be coconut, palm, or palm kernel oil, since the saturated vegetable oils are cheaper.

♦ "High in polyunsaturates." Manufacturers are not required by law to give the ratio of polyunsaturated fats to saturated fats, so you have to know your oils. The ones to go for are canola, corn, cottonseed, sunflower, safflower, soybean, or a combination of these.

♦ "Low-fat." In the case of dairy products this means that the product contains between .4 and 2 percent milk fat. With meat it means no more than 10 percent fat. For anything else, it means nothing.

♦ "Extra-lean" meat. No more than 5 percent fat—of the weight, not the calories.

♦ "Lean" meat. No more than 10 percent fat of the total weight.

♦ "Lower fat" meat. Contains 25 percent less fat of the total weight than usual.

SUGAR

In labelese "sugar" means sucrose, so a product that has no table sugar but is loaded with sorbitol, glucose, fructose, or any other *ose* word may legally be called "sugar-free." Be on the lookout for brown sugar, corn syrup, and honey.

♦ "Naturally sweetened." This means that the product has been sweetened with fruit or fruit juice.

SODIUM

♦ "Sodium-free." Fewer than 5 milligrams per serving.

♦ "Very low sodium." This means no more than 35 milligrams per serving.

♦ "Low sodium." A serving contains 140 milligrams or less.

♦ "Reduced sodium." The product contains 75 percent less sodium than usual.

♦ "Unsalted" or "no salt added." This means just what it says, but it does not mean that a product is low in sodium. Unsalted foods may still be very salty.

FIBER

There are no regulations about labeling fiber, so there are plenty of inappropriate "high fiber" labels out there, especially on cereals and soups.

♦ "Whole wheat." Ounce for ounce, enriched white bread and whole wheat bread are nutritionally very similar, but because white bread is made from refined flour, it has no fiber. Whole wheat bread does have fiber, but only if it's the Real McCoy; some breads labeled "wheat" are just white bread to which caramel coloring has been added. Look for the words "whole grain" or "whole wheat flour" at the beginning of the ingredients list.

♦ "Crude fiber." Means nothing.

MISCELLANEOUS

♦ "RDA." This stands for Recommended Daily Allowance, and it outlines what the U.S. government says are the various nutrients needed each day to maintain good health. These are ballpark figures, subject to change according to age and gender and whether you're pregnant or breastfeeding.

♦ "Enriched." Products that have lost nutrients during processing may have some of them replaced. When this happens (as it often does with bread), the product is referred to as enriched.

♦ "Fortified." When vitamins and minerals not commonly present in a product (cereal, for example) are added to it, it's called fortified.

♦ "Substitute." The product is nutritionally equivalent to the food it resembles.

♦ "Imitation." The product contains fewer vitamins, minerals, or other nutrients than the food it resembles.

♦ "Natural." When it's used to describe meat and poultry, it means that the product has been minimally processed and is free of artificial ingredients. When it's used to describe anything else, it means nothing. Many "natural" foods are highly processed, packed with fat and sugar, and loaded with artificial flavorings and preservatives.

♦ "Organic." Means nothing.

THE MATHEMATICS OF FOOD LABELS

To figure out the percentage of fat in a prepared food:

1   See how many calories are contained in one serving.
2   Check to see how many grams of fat are in one serving.
3   Multiply the number of grams of fat by nine, the number of calories in one gram of fat.
4   Divide that number by the total number of calories in a serving.

To work out the percentage of carbohydrates and protein, multiply the number of grams of carbohydrates or protein by four.

#11. WATCH OUT FOR THE LITTLE THINGS

Of course, there are hundreds of small ways to improve your diet. (If there weren't, women's magazines would soon go out of business.) These are some of our favorites.

♦ Get yourself a few kitchen gadgets: a gravy separator, a steamer, a nonstick pan, a hot-air popcorn popper, and a shredder (to make cheese go further).

♦ Switch to skim milk. This may take a while, since skim milk is an acquired taste. If you're used to whole milk, cut down to 2 percent, then to 1 percent, and eventually to skim. Some people add a tablespoon or two of nonfat dry milk to skim milk to give it more flavor.

♦ Start your meals with soup. Two of the most popular dishes on the

Ranch menu are the consommé and the gazpacho. The soups offer a flavorful low-cal, low-fat way to take the edge off an appetite. For best results eat soup with a spoon; drinking it from a mug makes it go too fast.

♦ Make peanut butter a meal. Peanut butter is high in calories and fat, but that doesn't mean you have to scratch it off your shopping list forever. You do have to think about it differently. Make a couple of tablespoons your protein source instead of a throw-away snack.

♦ Change your formula for salad dressing. Forget the old 4-to-1 ratio of oil to vinegar. If you must have oil in your dressing, work your way to a 3-to-1 ratio, then to 2-to-1, and eventually 1-to-1.

♦ Flavor your own yogurt. If you like flavored yogurts, you can cut down on sugar and fat by adding fresh fruit, such as sliced peaches or bananas or crushed berries, to plain nonfat yogurt. For even more flavor add a little vanilla or nutmeg.

♦ Learn to love angel food cake. A slice of angel food cake has 125 calories, fewer than half of the devil's food equivalent, and less than a gram of fat. Devil's food cake has about 5 grams of fat, and that's plain; with frosting it may contain as many as 15 grams of fat. Even with a fruit topping, angel food cake is still a caloric bargain.

♦ Fiddle with recipes. Try substituting water, juice, stock, or skim milk for fat. Make sauces by puréeing vegetables or fruits.

♦ Use nonfat yogurt instead of mayonnaise and sour cream. If you're serving it cold, you can use the yogurt as is. If you're heating it, mix in a tablespoon of flour per cup of yogurt to prevent it from separating.

♦ Use a nonstick pan for frying or sautéeing and instead of using butter try water, wine, stock, or even juice. Onions don't need to be sautéed in anything; since they're mostly water, they can be cooked in their own fluid.

♦ Learn ethnic cooking. The Chinese, Japanese, Italians, Thais, and Greeks have the right idea when they cook; their meals are usually long on carbohydrates and short on fat. Take a page out of their books.

♦ Slim down your tuna sandwich. Three ounces of tuna canned in oil have eleven grams of fat; the same amount canned in water has one gram of fat. Mix it with yogurt instead of mayonnaise.

♦ For a low-fat burger ask your butcher to trim the fat from a lean cut of meat and then grind it for you. Use three ounces of beef per burger and, to add the moisture you used to get from fat, mix in a little tomato juice and chopped onion before you broil it.

♦ Splurge on sherbet instead of ice cream. A half-cup of ice cream has seven grams of fat; a half-cup of sherbet has one.

♦ When you need a cookie fix, choose cookies that are relatively low in fat (ginger snaps, graham crackers, animal crackers, and fig newtons) and preferably not a hundred of them.

15

"I really thought that I could buy a package of cookies and eat just a few. First I took three and put the package away. Then I took four more and put it away again, this time on a higher shelf behind some pots and pans so that I couldn't get at it so easily. A half-hour later I dragged out the step-stool and helped myself to five more. After I finished those, I headed back to the kitchen and realized that I had completely lost control: I was obviously going to eat the entire two-pound bag of cookies. I thought about putting them in the freezer or throwing them in the trash, but I didn't think that would be enough. I finally did the only thing I knew would keep me from eating them. I put them under water."

The people enrolled in the Canyon Ranch "Managing Your Food Habits" seminar hear a lot of stories like that one, and most of them tell a few before they're through. Julie Kembel, who conducts the meeting, usually gets the ball rolling by explaining how and why she herself lost 55 pounds. As Julie tells her story—revealing how, for instance, she finally made the decision to lose weight the day she refused to take her coat off at work because she looked so awful—it becomes increasingly clear that the session is not really going to be about food. The subject at hand is *behavior*.

Yes, it is vitally important to eat the right things; we've just devoted a couple of lengthy chapters to explaining what those things are. However, there is much more to weight control than knowing saturated fats are bad and carbohydrates are good. In order to reach your desired weight and stay there, you have to change your eating habits. As we've said before (and will say again), the first step to changing behavior is understanding it. For the moment, then, let's

MANAGING YOUR EATING HABITS

leave the world of what we eat and talk about why we eat.

WHY WE EAT

If everyone ate only when he was hungry, there would be no Managing Your Food Habits seminars. Food does indeed satisfy hunger pains, but that's the least of its functions; almost everyone continues to eat long after his stomach is full. Food comforts the mouth as well as the stomach. As anyone who has ever had to live on liquids can tell you, we like to chew and swallow food; chewing and swallowing may actually be relaxing to the jaw muscles. But the part of the body where food really goes to work is the head.

If you're like most people with a weight problem, food helps you to cope, allowing you to step back from unpleasant circumstances and providing aid and comfort when you're feeling needy. Often when you think you're hungry, what you really are is tense, anxious, annoyed, or unhappy. You turn to food for relief, and indeed you often get it, at least temporarily; the act of eating is quite comforting, especially if it's a pint of something sweet and creamy. Then the guilt and depression kick in.

The only way many of us know how to take a break is to eat, even though it's the break we want, not the food. How many times, especially in the late afternoons or on weekends and holidays, when your energy level is low, have you turned to food for diversion when what you really needed was a little fun? When you're restless and tired, you need something to pick you up and pique your interest, and unless you have non-eating activities to turn to, you'll often get your entertainment from food.

One of the best ways to stop overeating is to find something else you like to do. Start a stamp collection, play solitaire, listen to language tapes, work in the garden, take up tap dancing or needlepoint, go to a movie, play with the dog, read a novel, jump rope—anything to distract you, relax you, and keep you from rummaging in the refrigerator. There are many better ways to manage stress than feeding it; learn some of them (see Chapter 17 for stress management and relaxation techniques).

Everybody uses food for different reasons and to varying degrees. Answering the following questions will help you understand your relationship with food. Don't overthink your answers; just write down your initial response to each of the questions.

As you probably guessed, there are no "right" and "wrong" answers to that questionnaire, and no real grade. What your answers should give you, however, is an increased awareness of when and why you are tempted to eat. Notice the groupings of numbers, particularly fives and sevens, and see what they tell you. Virtually everyone uses food as some sort of coping tool; if you can understand the nature of yours, you can begin to think about a replacement. Maybe the next time you find yourself staring into the refrigerator when you know you're not hungry, you'll have some idea why you're there.

This first set of questions is designed to help you identify many of your daily eating patterns. Please rate each according to your typical response, from never (1) to always (7).

NEVER ······· ALWAYS

I eat breakfast.	1 2 3 4 5 6 7
I eat lunch.	1 2 3 4 5 6 7
I eat dinner.	1 2 3 4 5 6 7
I snack in the mornings.	1 2 3 4 5 6 7
I snack in the afternoons.	1 2 3 4 5 6 7
I snack in the evenings.	1 2 3 4 5 6 7
I plan my snacks in advance.	1 2 3 4 5 6 7
I plan my meals in advance.	1 2 3 4 5 6 7
I eat until the food is gone.	1 2 3 4 5 6 7
I am a fast eater.	1 2 3 4 5 6 7
I eat while standing at the counter.	1 2 3 4 5 6 7
I take some of every food served to me.	1 2 3 4 5 6 7
I need second servings.	1 2 3 4 5 6 7
When eating several different food items on my plate, I "save the best for last."	1 2 3 4 5 6 7
I prepare the next bite of food on my fork while still chewing on the last bite.	1 2 3 4 5 6 7
I taste while cooking.	1 2 3 4 5 6 7
The kitchen is the first room I enter when I come into the house.	1 2 3 4 5 6 7
I eat in the car.	1 2 3 4 5 6 7
I eat while reading or watching TV.	1 2 3 4 5 6 7
I eat only when I am hungry.	1 2 3 4 5 6 7

Please rate the impact of each of the factors below on your typical overeating responses. Rate each factor, in general, from very little (1) to very much (7).

VERY LITTLE ··· VERY MUCH

The sight of food	1 2 3 4 5 6 7
The smell of food	1 2 3 4 5 6 7
The sound of cooking or someone eating	1 2 3 4 5 6 7
Suggestion (ads, TV/radio)	1 2 3 4 5 6 7
Food available (within easy reach)	1 2 3 4 5 6 7

Chart (*continued*)

VERY LITTLE ··· VERY MUCH

Pressure from other people	1	2	3	4	5	6	7
Other people's eating behaviors	1	2	3	4	5	6	7
Real hunger	1	2	3	4	5	6	7
Physical illness or discomfort	1	2	3	4	5	6	7
Menstrual cycle	1	2	3	4	5	6	7
Loneliness	1	2	3	4	5	6	7
Boredom	1	2	3	4	5	6	7
Fatigue	1	2	3	4	5	6	7
Frustration	1	2	3	4	5	6	7
Stress	1	2	3	4	5	6	7
Anger	1	2	3	4	5	6	7
Disappointment	1	2	3	4	5	6	7
Depression	1	2	3	4	5	6	7
Happiness	1	2	3	4	5	6	7
Personal reward	1	2	3	4	5	6	7
The need to punish myself, or get back at someone else	1	2	3	4	5	6	7
The need to pamper myself	1	2	3	4	5	6	7
During times when other things have gone well for me	1	2	3	4	5	6	7
During times when other things have gone badly for me	1	2	3	4	5	6	7
I have trouble controlling my eating:							
in the mornings	1	2	3	4	5	6	7
in the afternoons	1	2	3	4	5	6	7
in the evenings	1	2	3	4	5	6	7
during weekdays	1	2	3	4	5	6	7
during weekends	1	2	3	4	5	6	7
during holidays	1	2	3	4	5	6	7
in restaurants	1	2	3	4	5	6	7
in friends' homes	1	2	3	4	5	6	7
in my parents' home	1	2	3	4	5	6	7
in my own home when I have guests	1	2	3	4	5	6	7
in my own home when I am alone	1	2	3	4	5	6	7
after having wine or a cocktail	1	2	3	4	5	6	7
when wearing loosely fitting clothing	1	2	3	4	5	6	7
when wearing tightly fitting clothing	1	2	3	4	5	6	7
when wearing "grubbies"	1	2	3	4	5	6	7

BALANCE

If you're a typical dieter, the cycle probably goes something like this. For the first several days you're perfect, completely under control. You feel great, and you're very proud of yourself. Then you eat too much or the wrong thing one day, and you react by doing one of two things: you abandon all control and eat everything in sight, or you try to make up for your mistake by skipping a few meals. Either way, your response is wrong.

Ballet dancers return to first position between moves; the body is balanced on both feet and the arms are close in, which makes it easy to move into another position. Dieters should return to first position too. If you slip off your diet, return to your normal behavior. If a chicken sandwich is what you usually have for lunch, have it, even if you've put away half a dozen doughnuts for breakfast and you're not hungry. Returning to your usual regimen puts you back on an even keel and in control of your behavior. Dieting any other way is like having one foot on the scale and the other on a banana peel—one slip and you're flat on your back.

SETTING GOALS

One of the things most likely to throw you off balance is setting goals you can't reach. Short-term goals are best; if you want to lose 50 pounds altogether, you'll reach it only once if you think of the goal as 50 pounds. If you take it five pounds at a time, you can celebrate ten times before you're through. Very short-term goals—such as, "Today I'll eat only 1500 calories" or, "Tonight I won't eat before bedtime"—are excellent too. Long- or short-term, your goals should be realistic. There is no point in saying that you'll never touch cake again if you know that's just not possible.

Be patient. We're all familiar with creeping weight gain. It's time to think in terms of creeping weight loss. Most dieters want the longevity of a marathon at the speed of a sprint, forgetting that sprinters can't make it all the way through a marathon. You didn't put on all that weight in a few weeks, and there is no reason it should come off that fast.

In addition to being impatient many dieters have an all-or-nothing attitude when it comes to eating. Most of us are much too rigid in the demands we make on ourselves; we don't give ourselves any room in which to move around. We're good at letting go, but we're bad at letting up. Don't have just one plan. Just as most people have several exercise regimens—for instance, the maximum workout is running five miles, the moderate one calls for working out to an exercise tape, and the absolute minimum is doing 15 minutes of abdominals—you should give yourself some leeway when it comes to food. Ideally you'll reduce the calorie density of your food, reduce the volume, and reduce the frequency with which high-calorie foods are eaten, but if you can't do all three, you can at least choose one. Remember, some good behavior every day is better than none, and some good days are better than no good days.

PREPARING FOR SETBACKS

Julie Kembel tells a story about an overweight woman who had been trying to lose weight but was getting nowhere. The woman had a family reunion coming up, and she was really dreading it; one of her family's favorite things to do when they got together was to talk about who had gained the most weight since last time. The woman was pretty sure she was the unlucky winner, and she was also sure that if they started in on her, she would eat her way through the party and make matters even worse.

The woman decided that the best defense was a good offense. She bought a huge dress, five or six sizes too big, and stuffed her clothes with cotton. Then she walked into the party, took off her coat, showed her family her expanded new body, and beat them to the punch. *"I won,"* she announced.

The woman's stunt gave her a psychological edge and kept her from making the reunion a destructive experience. She put herself in charge. When you have setbacks—and you probably will—you need not go to the trouble of stuffing your clothes with cotton, but don't be too hard on yourself and do keep a positive attitude. Self-hate is a poor motivator. Don't let a disappointment throw you completely off track. Just return to first position and start again.

Don't be a slave to the scale, either. Instead of getting hung up on how much you weigh think about how much and how often you eat. Don't flog yourself for slip-ups; give yourself credit for the good choices you make.

NEW HABITS

The key to keeping motivation alive and reaching your goals is to make gradual changes that you can live with. If you really can't manage without chocolate or pizza, don't. If you can take mayonnaise and butter or leave them alone, leave them alone. Only you can decide what really matters to you. Making some sacrifices is inevitable, but if you ask yourself to give up too much, you'll rebel, probably by scrapping the whole plan.

The rest of this chapter describes some of the behavioral changes our guests have found to be most useful. Read it, think about it, and then make your own list, including the changes you think you can make. Revise the list often, crossing off the ones that have become second nature to you or those that you know you'll never manage and adding new challenges.

PLAN AHEAD

Get in the habit of checking your calendar at the beginning of the week and noting potentially risky situations, such as parties or late nights at the office. Pay attention to your body's rhythms. If you're ravenous every day at four o'clock, your body is probably telling you to give it an apple, a box of raisins, or a few crackers. If a meeting after work means an unusually late dinner, eat something before the meeting to keep you from getting too hungry.

SET A SMALLER TABLE

If you've ever served yourself at a salad bar, you know that the bigger the container is, the more salad you take, even if you don't even want all that lettuce. To control portion size try eating your meals from smaller bowls and plates and using smaller spoons and forks. Use measuring cups—the half-cup measure is about right—as serving spoons.

WEAR TIGHT CLOTHES

It's a lot easier to overeat when you're wearing baggy sweatpants or a roomy bathrobe than it is when your shirt is tucked into a pair of tight jeans or something with a real waistband. Wearing fitted clothes to the office may be why most of us don't stuff ourselves at breakfast and lunch.

SLOW DOWN

No matter what you're eating, it takes approximately 20 minutes from the time you begin to eat for your brain to tell your stomach that it's full. It stands to reason, then, that the longer you take to eat, the less likely you are to overeat. If you gobble that plate of cookies in two minutes flat, all you have are calories, guilt, and 18 minutes before you feel as if you've had enough. Practice eating more slowly and choose foods that buy you a little time: artichokes, hard shell crabs, soup, steamed clams, and salads.

Cut your food only as you need it and put down your utensils between bites. Don't load your fork again until you've swallowed.

Try nibbling instead of gobbling. Remember the last time a child gave you a bite of his candy bar? You would have taken a nice big bite, but the clever kid's fingers were in the way. Try to eat all of your food like that. Even if you're eating something bad for you, take it slow. Fast, guilty eating doesn't make the food less caloric; it just makes it less satisfying.

DON'T BE DISTRACTED

Because we eat all the time—in the car, in front of the television, in the office, on the run, in bed, practically everywhere but the shower—we associate far too many things with food. Eventually it may get so that we don't really enjoy those other activities unless we've got our mouths full. Get in the habit of eating without doing anything else, and only in the kitchen or dining room.

DON'T LET DINING OUT THROW YOU

Some weight-watchers think restaurants are a godsend—after all, you can have exactly what you want—but for others restaurant dining is murder on eating behavior. In Chapter 22 we discuss eating on the road at length.

DON'T MAKE EATING TOO INTERESTING

A certain monotony is good when it comes to eating. The more choices there are, the more you are inclined to eat; three foods seem to be the optimal number. Lavish buffets can be absolute killers. If you can't avoid them and you don't think you can trust yourself to make it through the line with only three foods on your plate, ask your spouse or a friend to fill your plate for you.

TAKE CHARGE AT HOME

Stop thinking of dinner parties as a showcase for elaborately prepared and highly caloric food and concentrate on good food and great company. Don't cook things for other people that you wouldn't eat yourself; you're just asking for trouble. Avoid family-style dining; serving bowls on the table encourage you to help yourself to seconds. When the meal is over, clear the table before coffee. Don't linger over tempting leftovers. In fact, give leftovers to your friends or stick them in the freezer right away, before you have a chance to polish them off. If you don't trust yourself to stay away from them and can't persuade someone to take them off your hands, pitch them.

AVOID TEMPTATION

Sometimes the only way to keep from eating certain foods is simply to keep them out of the house. Eat hard-to-control foods away from home in single portions. If you want a piece of pie, don't bring a pie home; go to a coffee shop and order a piece of pie. If you want ice cream, go out and have a cone; don't let a quart linger in the freezer. When you do have tempting foods in the house, keep them out of sight. Store leftovers in opaque hard-to-open containers or in paper bags and put them out of sight and out of reach.

DON'T EAT FROM A PACKAGE LARGER THAN YOUR HAND

Have you ever noticed that when you take a small serving from a large container, you feel cheated? After all, there is so much more where that came from. With some foods—nuts, for instance—there is no end until the container is empty. When you want a high-calorie snack, buy the snack size or single-serving bag. Don't buy tempting foods in units larger than you intend to consume. Never eat anything out of its original container. Unless you intend to eat a whole bag of cookies, don't leave the bag sitting around.

TAKING CHARGE

The urge to eat can sneak up on a person. Think back to the last time you were sitting in someone's living room, not a bit hungry as far as you knew, and your host set down a bowl of potato chips and some dip and a plate of cheese and crackers. The next thing you knew, you had blown your diet.

The next time you're about to eat something that you hadn't planned on, ask yourself, *Why this and why now?* Am I really hungry or am I angry, lonely, bored, afraid, or unhappy? Is there something else I can do besides eat? If not, will some other food, something more sensible, do the trick, or does it have to be a banana split? Then, taking full responsibility for your actions, do what you have to do.

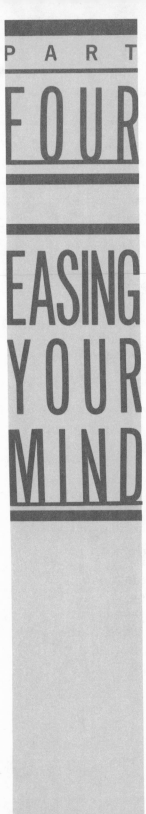

PART

FOUR

EASING YOUR MIND

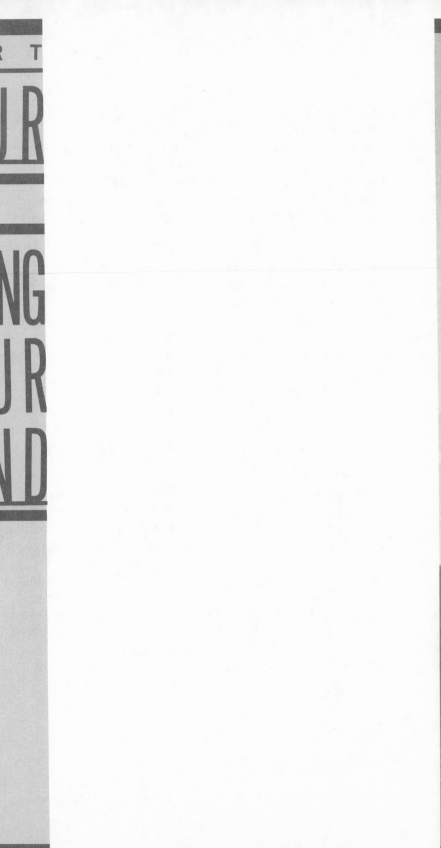

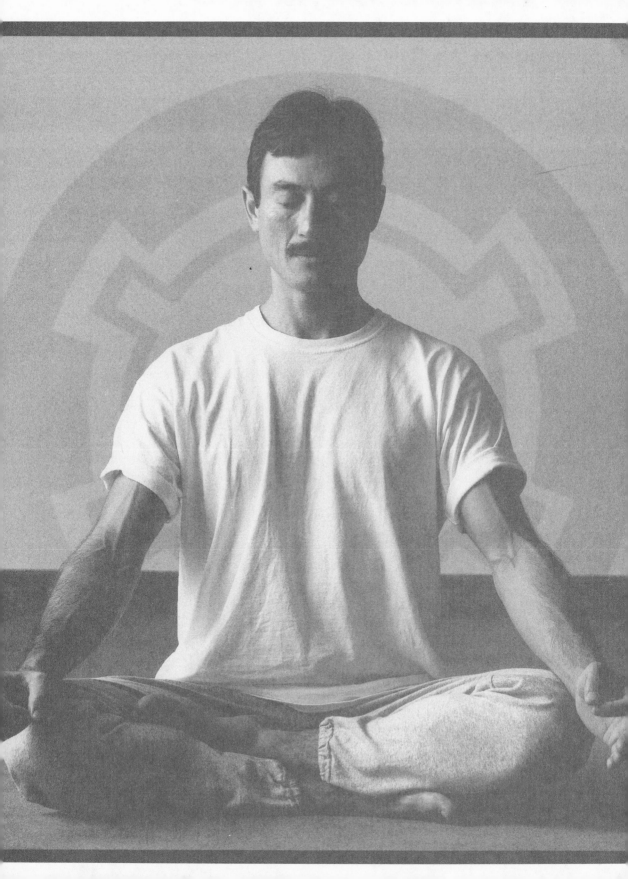

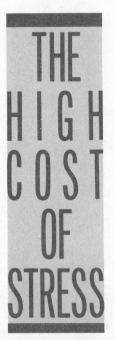

16

THE HIGH COST OF STRESS

Scenario #1: It's eleven o'clock at night, and you're sitting home alone, reading a good book and sipping a cup of tea. You hear a noise in the kitchen. The first thought that pops into your mind is that someone has broken into the house. Immediately you feel tense and scared. Your heart rate increases, your palms begin to sweat, you feel a little queasy, and your blood pressure goes up.

Scenario #2: It's eleven o'clock at night, and you're sitting home alone, reading a good book, and sipping a cup of tea. You hear a noise in the kitchen. You realize that it's the ice-maker. You keep reading.

These scenarios are used by former Canyon Ranch psychologist Kevan Schlamowitz to define stress. What happened in Scenario #1 is a variation on the fight-or-flight response that primitive man experienced when he was about to be attacked by a predator. When we sense danger, adrenaline is dumped into our bloodstream, triggering an increase in blood pressure, heart rate, blood flow, and metabolism. When we react to a perilous situation by running away or attacking our enemies, that adrenaline is used up and our bodies return to normal. However, when we don't fight back or run away, because the enemy is a deadline, a crazy boss, an unruly child, or even an ice-maker, the heart continues to pound, the stomach to churn, and the palms to sweat. In short, the energy that is "left over" is stress, and it's as dangerous an enemy as any predator.

One of the biggest changes in medical thinking over the last ten years or so is the recognition that stress is much more than an unpleasant side effect of our busy, difficult lives; the fact is, there is a physiological component to stress that can literally kill us.

Of course, everything that is arousing to the system is stressful to it in some way, and in small doses stress can be harmless, even stimulating. Many people find that they work particularly well under pressure, becoming more creative and more efficient. Others find the challenge of short-term stress, the kind you get from dodging rush-hour traffic, skiing a rough course, or making a difficult presentation, downright exhilarating. Long-term stress is something else again. It can exact a heavy emotional and physical toll, and it often has a debilitating effect on your behavior.

Americans consume about 16000 tons of aspirin, 5 billion tranquilizers, 3 billion amphetamines, and 3 billion barbiturates every year. It is estimated that more than two-thirds of all visits to the family doctor are caused by stress or have some stress-related component. According to a 1988 *Newsweek* magazine article, the cost of stress, including such factors as absenteeism and stress-related compensation claims, is now about $150 billion a year in this country. Clearly, we are a nation under stress.

THE SYMPTOMS OF STRESS

One of the major problems of stress is that it is very difficult to measure it in any precise way. Biofeedback is one measuring tool, of course, and there are questionnaires and psychological tests that provide some general insights. However, the single most reliable way of knowing you're suffering from stress is examining how you feel. Some of the most common symptoms of stress are headaches, tension, anxiety, sweating, loss of self-confidence, fear, panic, irritability, frustration, and a knot in the stomach that won't go away. You may also find yourself worrying all the time and unable to concentrate or enjoy life. In some cases you're overwhelmed with a frequent desire to cry or run away.

These emotional symptoms may lead to unpleasant behavioral changes too, such as crying, yelling, nail-biting, forgetfulness, teeth-grinding, and a change in appetite, sleep patterns, and sexual functioning. When you're under stress, you may become accident-prone, unable to work, or increasingly dependent on tobacco, alcohol, drugs, and food.

Even if they are not obvious, the manifestations of stress are felt in virtually every part of the body:

♦ Cardiovascular system. Stress may lead to high blood pressure, coronary artery distress, arrhythmia, and stroke.

♦ Muscular system. Stress can cause tension headaches and muscle-contraction backaches.

♦ Locomotor system. Stress contributes to the incidence of rheumatoid arthritis and other related inflammatory diseases of the connective tissue.

♦ Respiratory and allergic disorders. Asthma, hay fever, and other allergies may be brought on by stress.

♦ Immune system. When some people endure prolonged periods of stress, they produce fewer white blood cells, which means that their resistance to disease is lowered.

♦ Gastro-intestinal system. Stress can bring on ulcers, irritable bowel syndrome, diarrhea, nausea, and colitis.

♦ Genito-urinary system. Stress has a role in diuresis, sexual dysfunction, and menstrual problems.

♦ Skin. Stress may cause eczema, neurodermatitis, and acne.

ARE YOU OVERSTRESSED?

According to the National Mental Health Association, anxiety and tension are essential functions of living, but there is such a thing as too much of a good thing. If you answer yes to most of the following questions, you may have a serious problem with stress.

1 Do minor problems throw you for a loop?
2 Do you find it hard to get along with people with whom you used to be compatible?
3 Does nothing seem to give you pleasure?
4 Are you unable to stop thinking about your problems?
5 Do you feel distrustful and suspicious much of the time?
6 Do you feel trapped and/or inadequate?

WHAT CAUSES STRESS?

Canyon Ranch Health Services Director Dan Baker says that stress is the reaction you have to the difference between what you hope for and expect in life and what reality delivers. For instance, if you hope and expect that your children will be brilliant scholars and Olympic athletes and they turn out to be C students who can't walk and chew gum at the same time, you will probably experience stress. If the kids flunk out of school and steal hubcaps, you'll be even more stressed.

There are other, equally valid ways of defining stress, but everyone who defines it agrees on one thing: stress doesn't come only from outside; it comes from within as well.

One of the most common stress-producing mind games we play involves "polarized thinking," which is a fancy way of saying that to many of us everything is black and white, good or bad, success or failure, all or nothing. If you smoke one cigarette, you may as well smoke the carton. If you have one cookie, you've blown your diet. If you quit exercising for a week, you may as well give it up forever. This kind of thinking is enormously, and unnecessarily, stressful.

Here are a few other examples.

DISTORTED BELIEFS

Let's go back to the two scenes we described at the beginning of this chapter, when you were sitting alone and you heard a noise. When you thought the noise was a burglar, you were terrified, but when you thought it was the ice-maker, you were completely relaxed. So basically it was not the noise that caused you to be upset; it was your perception of the noise. How you look at an event largely determines the significance of it. If you believe that something is a disaster, you'll feel bad about it. If you regard it as good news, you'll feel good. It may sound a little trite to say it, but it's nonetheless true: things don't upset you; *you* upset you.

Naturally there are times of genuine emergency or crisis in everyone's life that cannot be willed away by the power of positive thinking. Even then, however, you can exercise some control over the amount of stress you experience. If a tidal wave were about to engulf your city, you would, of course, be upset and afraid, but that doesn't mean you have to become hysterical. You can choose to stay calm, and in fact you'd probably be much better off if you did. It's up to you. You have a great deal more control over your thoughts and emotions than you realize, provided you behave rationally.

Kevan Schlamowitz used to tell the story about a young newlywed who was having her first dinner party. She wanted to make something special, so she asked her mother for her pot roast recipe. Her mother told her that the first thing she must do is cut the end of the roast off before putting it in the pan. When the new bride asked her mother why that step was necessary, the older woman said she didn't know, really; that was the way her mother always did it. Still curious, the young woman asked her mother's mother the same question and got the same answer: the grandmother learned the method from her own mother. More determined than ever to get the answer to her question, the bride visited her great-grandmother and begged her for the cooking secret. Why, she asked, was it necessary to cut the end off the roast before putting it in the oven? The answer was simple: the great-grandmother had never had a roasting pan big enough for the whole roast, so she had to cut the end off.

That's how many distorted beliefs get started. At one point there was a reason for certain actions—and a good reason at that—but it has long since lost its meaning. Many of us are governed by beliefs that make no more sense than Great-Grandma's pot roast recipe.

CATASTROPHIZING

Picture a man and a woman sitting under a tree on a sunny afternoon. They've been picking flowers, and they're ready to have their lunch, which they carried in a picnic basket filled to the brim. Nearby is a small, playful dog with a ball in his mouth.

Now let's play the "What If?" game. Think of all the terrible things that might happen to the couple.

What if they're sitting on an anthill?
What if it rains?
What if lightning strikes?
What if they're allergic to flowers?
What if they get sunburned?
What if there are snakes in the grass?
What if they get grass stains?
What if the dog runs away?
What if they get food poisoning?

The exercise may seem silly, but the fact is that many of us play this game, or something very like it, all the time. When we travel, we wonder, "What if the plane crashes?" or "What if they lose my luggage?" When we have a headache, we think, "What if it's a brain tumor?" We look into the future and worry and spend emotional energy on something that hasn't happened yet and probably won't.

OVERSPENDING

A man sees a pair of running shoes he likes in a store window and asks the clerk how much they cost. The clerk tells the customer that the price is 50 dollars. The shopper pays the clerk 100 dollars and leaves the store.

Yes, this scene is even sillier than the "What if?" game, but it too is an example of the games many of us play with our emotions. Hardly a day goes by that we don't spend a hundred dollars' worth of emotional energy on a 50-dollar problem. Another way Kevan Schlamowitz likes to look at stress is as the overspending of emotions.

Like money, emotional energy is valuable and limited, so you don't want to waste it any more than you want to squander your hard-earned cash. If it helps, think of your emotions as dollar bills. Keep in mind that every day you have a certain number of emotional dollars to spend. If you waste them by fuming in traffic jams or complaining loudly in slow-serving restaurants, you'll run out of "money" in a hurry, and the penalty for going broke is getting sick. There is a physical price to pay for any emotion.

Of course, life is not a retail shoe store, and daily events don't come with price tags. How you label the world determines how you interact with the world. Only you can figure out the price of the things that happen in your own life, and if your perception is sometimes not accurate—when it's the ice-maker instead of the burglar, for instance—you waste a lot of emotion.

The point here is not to tell you never to worry or get angry or emotional; it's to say that you should worry only as much as something is worth and get angry only if anger helps you. Conserve your emotions the same way you conserve your money.

"HOT REACTORS"

Most people are familiar with the terms Type A and Type B in regard to people's behavior and the incidence of heart disease. Type A behavior is characterized by impatience, hostility, and explosiveness of speech. Type B people tend to be passive and relaxed. Both types are identified by their observed behavior, which may or may not have anything to do with the physical realities. That is, Type A people may be "hyper," but that doesn't mean they necessarily have high blood pressure or are headed for a heart attack.

A new term has come on the scene that has considerably more significance in this area: hot reactor. A hot reactor is someone whose blood pressure becomes inordinately high when he experiences mental or emotional stress. (At the Ranch we give a series of three tests—a video game, a mental task, and a physical challenge—to identify hot reactors.) About 70 percent of all hot reactors are likely to develop chronic hypertension within three years, and hot reactors may be at greater risk of heart attack or stroke than cool reactors.

Only about one out of five people with normal resting blood pressure readings is a hot reactor, and the condition doesn't have to be permanent. With treatment and behavioral changes hot reactors can train themselves to cool down.

THE FIRST STEP

One of Dan Baker's favorite stories is about a businessman who was traveling in Saudi Arabia several years ago. As he was being shown around the city of Riyadh one day, he saw two brand-new Mercedes collide head-on at an intersection. Both drivers leaped out and ran toward each other, and the man fully expected to see an old-fashioned fistfight. The unfortunate drivers did confront each other but not with their fists. Instead they embraced and began talking animatedly, smiling all the while. The confused businessman asked his interpreter for an explanation.

"Well, you see, sir," he was told, "everything that happens here is considered to be the will of God. The men are saying how wonderful it is that Allah arranged for them to meet."

Life throws many things at us—head-on collisions in our brand-new Mercedes, domestic strife, impossible deadlines, and ice-makers that sound like burglars—and sometimes it seems that the only truly sane reaction is to get an ulcer or light up a cigarette or grind your teeth or have a nice big bowl of ice cream. But none of those things really makes you feel better, and even more to the point, none of those things makes whatever is causing you stress go away. Even if it did make them go away, there will be others to take their place. The only way to fight stress is to learn to manage and control it. In the next chapter we'll talk about specific ways of doing just that.

17

You've always known that carrying around extra weight is bad for your health; now you know that carrying extra stress can be just as bad, maybe worse. To be truly well you must do more than eat right and exercise. You have to learn to manage stress.

The American Dream, with its emphasis on success, achievement, and self-reliance, is a veritable stress factory. These days it's almost impossible to live your life without some sort of stress. If you can't avoid stress, you can manage it, but like every other facet of wellness, stress management requires your participation and commitment. You have to be just as committed to your relaxation as you are to eating right and getting regular exercise. Managing stress means managing yourself.

We've been trying to get that message across for years, but only recently have people really begun to pay attention to stress. When Canyon Ranch first opened, only about 5 percent of our guests were interested enough in the "head stuff" we offered to follow the little bird tracks up the hill to our Behavioral Services department. Today, nine years later, more than 25 percent of the guests at least explore some form of stress management (today they do it in the new Health and Healing Center next to the Spa). Some of them have simply worked their way up; having learned about diet and exercise, they are now ready to move on to the next step. Others are there because they have specific problems to solve and need some new tools to help them. Still others are just curious or eager to try something new.

Many of the guests we see are accustomed to coping with the stresses of the day by "burning them up" with vigorous exercise. They are surprised to learn that while exercise is undoubtedly beneficial, it is not the same thing as relaxation.

PREVENTING AND MANAGING STRESS

Easing stress does not mean running in place until you've used up all your adrenaline and you're too exhausted to be tense and nervous; it means teaching yourself to relax.

Ideally, easing the mind will involve something that engages the mind. Getting a massage and soaking in a hot tub are perfectly acceptable relaxation techniques, but some even better ones are progressive relaxation, yoga, meditation, autogenic suggestion (in which you use your mind to control your heartbeat, breathing, and blood pressure), reading, working crossword puzzles, even playing cards or chess. Hobbies, such as collecting shells, bird-watching, or photography, can be excellent stress-relievers, too.

TAKING TIME TO PREVENT STRESS

In most of the remainder of this chapter we'll explore in detail several of the most effective stress management techniques. Before we get into those, however, here are some general techniques with which you should become familiar. They were specifically designed with the busy executive in mind, but there is no reason that they can't be adapted to everyone else.

♦ Stop thinking that the longer you work, the more productive you will be. Realize that there is a point of diminishing returns. Take that hour when you're not really being very productive and use it to recharge your batteries.

♦ If your schedule is impossibly tight, write in some personal time, even if it's only 15 minutes between meetings. Use that time for deep breathing, meditation, progressive relaxation, or giving yourself a neck and shoulder massage. (See Chapter 20 for more about self-massage.)

♦ Understand what happens to you when you get tired. If you're like most people, you're more likely to crave junk food and cigarettes or drink too much coffee when you're fatigued. If you can't avoid these periods of fatigue, learn to substitute deep breathing or other relaxation techniques until the unhealthy cravings pass.

♦ Every hour drink a glass of water and take ten deep breaths. To monitor yourself keep a large pitcher of water on your desk and make sure it's empty by the time the workday is over.

♦ Learn to recognize when your body is in a "fight or flight" mode. Some people feel it in their neck, their hands, or their stomachs. Others get very tired quite suddenly. When you feel these symptoms coming on, be ready to act on them.

♦ Don't tune out your body. The ability to think about only the project at hand is perceived to be a great asset, for obvious reasons, but getting totally lost in your work can be hazardous to your health. If you're oblivious to the demands of your body, you may miss some important messages; then all of a sudden you'll end up with a throbbing headache or a painful twinge in your back or an ulcer that is killing you.

♦ Practice "stress prevention." For example, if waiting in line drives you mad, never go anywhere without something to read. If missing a meal makes you want to eat everything in sight, have an apple or a box of raisins in your briefcase or handbag at all times. Sometimes stress is caused by the feeling that someone else is in control. Having an alternative behavior allows you to reestablish control over a situation.

THE TECHNIQUES

At Canyon Ranch we believe that the best way to manage stress is through cognitive behavioral therapy, which is a lofty way of saying that we teach people that they can change the way they feel by changing the way they think about things. Feelings are preceded by thoughts, so by controlling the thoughts, you can control your feelings. If you don't regard an event as a catastrophe, the thinking goes, you will not get an ulcer over it.

That all sounds simple enough, but of course, it isn't. Changing the way we regard the world doesn't come easily; after all, we've taken a lifetime to develop our thought patterns, even if they are a little distorted, and we can't make them disappear overnight. Certainly we can't make them disappear without a little help.

We don't expect you to fight stress alone. Here are some of the most useful tools we know of to help you along. Just as you must learn to identify what it is that pushes your "panic" button, you must decide which of the following techniques gives you the relief you need.

BREATHING

Of all the relaxation techniques we recommend, there is one that never gets a bad review from anyone: breathing. Breathing exercises are easy to do, the benefits are immediate and obvious, they don't take very long, and they don't make you feel too silly. In general, the deeper your breathing is, the more relaxed you will be. Most people are shallow breathers; they don't take advantage of the pleasure that comes from filling their lungs with air. At the very least, you should be breathing deeply for a few minutes a couple of times a day.

Here are a few specific breathing techniques.

RELAXING BREATH

Inhale deeply through your nose, filling your chest cavity and then your abdomen. Hold it for a second or two, then exhale gently, releasing the air from the abdomen first, then from the chest. Repeat several times.

COOLING BREATH

Try this on a really hot day.

Roll your tongue as if you were wrapping it around a pencil. Inhale and exhale through your mouth several times. Feel how the air coming over your tongue seems to cool the respiratory system.

CLEANSING BREATH

To recharge your circulatory system, breathe in and out of your nose rapidly for about three minutes.

ABDOMINAL BREATHING

Close your eyes and concentrate. Breathe in deeply through your nose, letting your abdominal muscles expand as far as they can go. Exhale through your mouth, letting your abdominals contract; empty your body completely. Say, *"Haaa"* as you exhale. Repeat several times.

MIDDLE CHEST BREATHING

This exercise is very relaxing; it may even put you to sleep if you do it long enough.

Breathe in through your nose, allowing your middle chest to open and expand. Exhale through your mouth, slowly and gradually (say, *"Haaa"* again), letting your middle chest become smaller and tighter. Repeat several times.

UPPER CHEST BREATHING

Inhale through your nose. As you take in oxygen, lift your breastbone toward the ceiling, as if the weight of the world has been lifted from your chest. When you exhale, through your mouth, lower your breastbone back onto your chest, almost as if it's collapsing. Repeat several times.

FULL BODY BREATHING

Inhale through your nose slowly, letting the air fill first your abdomen, then your middle chest, and finally your upper chest. Focus on your breathing. Then, very slowly, breathe out (say, *"Haaa"*), letting the air leave the abdomen first, then the middle chest, and finally the upper chest. Repeat several times.

ALTERNATE NOSTRIL BREATHING

In most people one nostril usually dominates, so it's good practice to give the other a chance once in a while. Alternate nostril breathing has been known to lower blood pressure and slow the heartbeat. This breathing exercise is a little tricky, but if you do it smoothly and quietly, it can be very soothing.

Put the thumb of your right hand on your right nostril and use the ring finger of that hand to cover your left nostril. Keeping your mouth closed all the time, close off your right nostril and breathe in through your left nostril to the count of four; then close off the left and exhale through the right nostril to the count of eight. Repeat several times. Then switch sides: close off the left and breathe in from the right; close off the right and breathe out from the left. After doing it several times, switch again.

BREATHING TO FIGHT TEMPTATION

When the urge to smoke or drink or eat something you shouldn't comes over you, try this technique. Pucker your lips (think about eating a bitter lemon) and breathe in through your mouth as if you were breathing through a straw. Take the air in slowly, savoring the breath, and when you have taken in as much as you can hold, exhale through your puckered lips. Do this breathing exercise for at least 90 seconds.

PROGRESSIVE RELAXATION

If you could spend 10 to 20 minutes a day, every day, clearing your head and tuning out your environment, chances are you could beat your stress problem. One of the best ways to spend that time is doing progressive relaxation. This process definitely takes some getting used to, but it's extremely effective as a stress-reliever. Here's how to do it.

Wearing comfortable clothes and no shoes, lie down on a flat surface and breathe slowly and evenly. (If it's impossible to lie down, you can do this sitting in a chair.) As you inhale, scan a muscle area, identifying any trouble spots: aches, pains, tightness, whatever. As you exhale, let the pain and tension go from that area. Then move on to the next region. Start with your head and work your way down to the face, neck, shoulders, arms, chest, stomach, back, legs, and feet. Spend a moment scanning and then letting tension go from each part of your body. When you're finished with your entire body, rest for a few moments before you get up. (You can do this in 20 minutes or less.) Concentrate on remembering what it feels like when your body is without tension. Make it your goal to be able to summon up that feeling at will.

MEDITATION

Many of us are great at being lazy, but very few are good at being still; we have no idea of how good it can feel. Being completely still is what meditation is really all about.

It is more than that, of course. Once you know how to do it, meditation can help you concentrate, allow you to solve problems and become more creative, and make it easier for you to escape the tensions of the day. It is wonderful for relieving stress. It's not easy to learn how to meditate (the hardest thing about it is keeping your mind from wandering) but with practice everyone can eventually get the hang of it. The more you meditate, the easier it gets, and the deeper your stillness will become. Eventually your body and mind will actually come to crave the meditative state.

Most people who meditate regularly have strong feelings about when, where, and how they do it—always at sunrise sitting on a soft cotton blanket and staring at a silver clock, for example—but there are no absolutes in meditation. A quiet environment, free from distractions, is highly recommended, and so is a certain consistency of time and place. If you get used to meditating at the same time every day, such as every morning when you get up or right after lunch every day or just before going to sleep, you will find it easier to reach the meditative state. If you're serious about meditating, you'll do it every day, for 15 to 30 minutes at a time.

Some like to turn meditation into a full-fledged ritual: they shower or bathe beforehand, light candles and incense, arrange cut flowers to focus on, and wear only loose, flowing robes made of natural fibers. All of these extras can make meditation a lovely experience, but none of it is necessary; all you really need are comfort and quiet. You can even meditate in your office, provided you won't be disturbed.

MEDITATING ON YOUR BREATHING

There are many different ways of meditating, but all of them require that you meditate *on* something: a word, an object, or even a thought. One of the most elemental forms of meditation uses focused breathing as that object. This exercise, which creates deep mental and physical relaxation, is especially helpful in stress management.

♦ Get completely comfortable. If possible, sit on the floor or on the bed with your back straight and your legs crossed at the ankles. Make sure that there are no distractions in the room. Take two deep breaths.

♦ Focus your eyes on a spot and keep them trained there throughout this exercise. (If you close your eyes, you may fall asleep.) Breathe normally and think about your breath.

♦ Begin counting your breath cycles; one cycle consists of an inhalation and an exhalation. Count by saying, "Inhale one, relax . . . Inhale two, relax" to yourself. When you reach ten, return to one and start counting again. Do at least 30 breaths per session. If you lose track, return to one and start counting again.

♦ When you're finished, take a deep, refreshing breath.

YOGA

Anyone who looks at fitness instructor Mary Margaret Walmer finds it very hard to believe that she's 65 years old. Anyone who takes her Advanced Yoga class finds it absolutely impossible to believe that Mary Margaret used to be virtually crippled; 20 years ago her back was in such bad shape that she couldn't even stand up straight. Today if there were a "Best Posture" contest at Canyon Ranch, she would win hands down. And she owes it all to yoga.

Yoga does a lot more than give you good posture. It improves your flexibility and your strength, and it has a beneficial effect on the tendons, muscles, joints, ligaments, bones, nervous system, even the skin. Yoga can be immensely helpful in relieving chronic backache, tension, and stress. (Many people fall asleep during the relaxation part of our yoga classes.) There's a spiritual element to yoga as well. The precision of the movements, the necessity of placing every part of your body carefully and precisely, forces you to concentrate and get completely in touch with your body.

As little as 15 to 30 minutes of yoga a day can make a huge difference in the way you feel, and one of the best things about it is that virtually anyone can do it, with the help and guidance of a qualified teacher. If you would like to give yoga a try, check with a local college or university, the YMCA, or one of your community centers to see if they offer yoga instruction. If they do have teachers, ask for references and credentials. Sit in on a class or two before you enroll officially. Establishing a rapport with the instructor is desirable in all classes, but in yoga it's essential. Don't stay in a class you don't like.

HYPNOTHERAPY

A man walked into V. V. Hughes's office one day for a four P.M. hypnotherapy session. He had just come from a three o'clock Men's Stretch class, and he had a massage scheduled for five. "I'm here to quit smoking," he said, glancing at his watch. "How long is this going to take?"

If only it were that easy.

That "quick fix" element of hypnotherapy is only one of the many myths and misunderstandings that surround the practice. Most of the others stem from sitcom visions of hypnosis, in which the person being hypnotized stares at a swinging watch for a while, goes into a deep trance, and spends the rest of the show quacking like a duck or imagining that his pants are on fire whenever he hears the word "Chicago." The only hypnosis cliché that is true is that hypnosis requires a willing subject; if you don't want to be hypnotized, it won't happen.

Hypnotherapy, which is the name given to the therapeutic use of hypnosis, does not require going into a deep trance or losing control. It does involve letting go of all tension and allowing your mind to become calm. Your body may "go to sleep," but your mind becomes fully aware. When you are in this state of relaxed awareness, both the conscious and subconscious levels of your mind are more receptive to communication from an outside source. This state of heightened suggestibility is a fertile environment for processing information in a very sharp, focused way. Under hypnosis you can be creative, solve problems, and receive wisdom and inspiration. You can also plant the seeds of new behavior so as to achieve certain goals you set for yourself.

In describing the process of hypnotherapy we might do well to use an appropriate analogy for the computer age: reprogramming. To put it as simply as possible, hypnotherapy allows you to erase old programs of behavior and introduce new ones. Often the first step is an "uncovering" process, in which the therapist encourages the subject to find out why those original programs are in place—why, for instance, you keep overeating even though you know better or why you can't quit smoking even though you know it may well kill you. That information then allows you to know what new messages most need to be sent to your subconscious mind to bring about the desired change in behavior. Once you're in a suggestible state and have explored the motives behind your behavior, you can begin to rehearse some new behavior. In that suggestible state you are able to maximize the effect of those new images you rehearse: of you not smoking or you eating carrots instead of ice cream.

For instance, if you recall that as a child you were often told to be a "good" girl or boy and eat everything on your plate, and now as an overweight adult you feel compelled to finish everything that is put in front of you, you may need to reprogram, telling yourself that you can be "good" without cleaning your plate. In addition to verbal messages you are encouraged to create mental images of yourself as you follow through with your new behavior (pushing your plate away even though there is food still on it) or accomplish your goals (weight reduction). Hypnotherapy helps you change the way you think about yourself and reprogram your thoughts so that they correspond with your idea of who you want to be and how you want to behave.

V. V. Hughes says that hypnotherapy wouldn't work at all if it were not for one very important fact: everyone has the solution to his own problems within himself. Deep down we all know best what will relax us, energize us, motivate us, and help us work out our various neuroses. What's more, everyone has the potential for being helped by hypnosis; it's a natural state, and it has a wide range of application. People who are typically helped are people who want to break or modify habits, especially smoking, drinking, drugs, and overeating, or who want to do something about stress, sleep disorders, phobias, or pain.

If you're interested in trying hypnotherapy, you might ask a medical physician or a psychologist to recommend someone to you. If you end up turning to the Yellow Pages, ask potential therapists for references and credentials. Keep in mind that no two hypnotherapists conduct a session in exactly the same way, so you must find one who makes you comfortable and understands your needs. He or she may be guiding you through some rocky shoals, and you have to be willing to follow with trust.

BIOFEEDBACK

Your pupils are dilated, you're bathed in sweat, your heart is racing, there's a knot in your stomach, and you can feel your blood pressure climbing. In the old days all this would mean that you were being chased by a wild boar. Today it means you're giving a speech or running 10 minutes late for your dentist appointment. Stressful events produce strong emotions, which produce physical responses. Many of these responses are controlled by the sympathetic nervous system, the network of nerve tissue that helps the body meet emergencies.

It's those physical responses that are at the core of the relaxation therapy called biofeedback. If you've ever taken your temperature or measured your heart rate or blood pressure, you've used a form of biofeedback; you've let your body "feed back" information to you about how it was feeling at the time. Biofeedback is a treatment technique in which people are trained to improve their health by using signals from their own bodies. In a way, biofeedback lets you see and hear activity inside your own body.

Unlike the other relaxation tools we've discussed so far, biofeedback requires some hardware. Sensitive electronic equipment is used to measure changes in your internal physiology. During a biofeedback session changes in blood flow, nervous system arousal, and muscle tension are displayed as they happen. The method is noninvasive, using electrodes and a thermometer attached to the surface of the skin. The therapist helps you to understand the responses on the computer screen and makes suggestions based on the patterns that are displayed.

Biofeedback monitors a biological process that would be difficult, perhaps even impossible, for the subject to detect any other way. It's one thing to think that you are relaxed. It's another to have the evidence right in front of your eyes. By monitoring your performance in a whole new way, biofeedback helps you to identify stress-producing factors that you probably didn't even know were there. It also provides a vivid reminder that the brain is related to the body. When you see what happens to the monitoring device when you think about the argument you had with your kids, you realize all too well that emotional problems have physical responses.

Biofeedback doesn't actually do anything to you; it's an educational tool, one you can use for self-exploration. What do you do with all of your new-found knowledge? Almost anything. Some people get so good at it that they can slow their heart rate, decrease or increase their blood pressure, halt the muscle spasms that cause pain, and even modify their breathing and oxygen consumption. Biofeedback helps you control and manage stress, and it can also be very useful in treating a variety of ailments, among them asthma, insomnia, migraines and other headaches, tinnitus (ringing in the ears), chest pain, epilepsy, gastrointestinal disorders, high and low blood pressure, and Raynaud's disease, which affects the circulatory system. Physical therapists sometimes use biofeedback in the rehabilitation of stroke victims; it helps them get back in touch with their paralyzed muscles.

Biofeedback doesn't offer a quick fix any more than hypnotherapy and meditation do. Becoming proficient at it requires effort, practice, and time. It can be frustrating at times, particularly for people who are accustomed to being in control; they get annoyed when they can't get the needle to move or the bell to ring on cue. It's well worth the effort, though, especially when you are practiced enough to use the technique without the machine.

Many people are leery of biofeedback (Ranch biofeedback director Mary Deits has considered hanging a sign on her door that reads, "Skeptics

Welcome") but a session or two usually makes believers of all our guests. If you would like to try biofeedback, be sure that your biofeedback administrator (who may be a physician, a psychologist, a psychiatrist, a nurse, a social worker, or a physical therapist) is properly trained. Check the trainer's credentials with the Biofeedback Society of America, 4301 Owen Street, Wheatridge, Colorado 80033.

MindFitness

Remember those times when everything seemed to "click," when your work was going well, you were incredibly happy, and life suddenly seemed to fall into place? If you were able to measure the activity of your brain at those moments, you would probably discover that you were generating high levels of what scientists call alpha brain waves.

Alpha waves, one of the four kinds of brain wave patterns that scientists have identified, are associated with deep states of relaxation, creativity, imagination, and the experience of physical, emotional, and mental well-being. (The others are beta, theta, and delta. Beta is our normal waking state, theta is the relaxed state just before we fall asleep, and delta is deep sleep.)

Suppose you could have that alpha experience on a daily basis. What if it were possible to learn how to gain command of all four types of brain waves, and their associated physical, mental, and emotional states, so that you could create and enhance those moments at will?

With MindFitness you can. Now through sophisticated brain wave feedback technology—going biofeedback one better—and highly specialized mind management training almost anyone can learn how to activate those alpha waves on command. By teaching us how to generate and increase the alpha waves, the ones that make us feel relaxed, creative, energetic, and happy, MindFitness can help us work at optimum performance at will.

HOW IT WORKS

Sitting comfortably in a darkened room, you wear a sensor headset through which you listen to musical tones that are being generated by your own brain waves. The tones vary as your thoughts skip from one to another. As you listen to the feedback and receive periodic numerical scores, you begin to learn how to increase alpha waves purely through the power of your own mind. By experimenting with specific thoughts, daydreams, and blank moments, you learn precisely what causes your alpha scores to rise and fall. After several sessions it becomes easier to reach the alpha state. Eventually you can do it without the machine, whenever and wherever you want.

In addition to the immediate electronic feedback you later review a computer analysis of the actual quantities of specific brain waves you generated. A trainer guides you before and after each feedback session to help you understand what is happening to you and suggest ways that your new knowledge can help you.

WHAT IT'S GOOD FOR

One man came to the Ranch with dangerously high blood pressure. An aggressive, hard-driving executive, he had had two heart attacks and a triple bypass surgery operation, and four months later his recovery was not going well. He could barely get around without help. He was heavily medicated, but still his blood pressure hovered up around 150. After MindFitness training his blood pressure was down to 114 without medication. A month later he was on skis.

Then there was the 34-year-old policewoman who had lived with immense pain for seven years, until finally she was completely disabled. Clinically depressed, she attempted suicide. When she arrived at the Ranch for MindFitness training, she was bitter, angry, and hostile, and her list of physical and mental complaints had about 40 items on it. For two days she cried nonstop, complaining of pain and dizziness and despairing of ever getting well. By the end of MindFitness she was a completely changed woman, joyful, optimistic, and energetic. Much of her pain was gone, and she had a new lease on life. She went back to school to work on a new career. Her depression score dropped 43 percent, from "maximally disturbed" to normal.

Not all of the changes that MindFitness can bring about have "Movie of the Week" potential like those two, but the effects can be and usually are very impressive. Some of the other physical and psychological responses are:

◆ Greatly reduced stress. Being in an alpha state actually makes your blood pressure go down, a great boon to hypertensives. People have also had success preventing and getting rid of tension headaches. MindFitness can help hard-driving overachievers learn to calm down.

◆ Increased productivity and heightened creativity. Have you ever noticed that ideas pop into your head when they are least expected? Sometimes when you "switch off" your mind, you begin to use your intuition, to gain insights and make connections between things that you might not otherwise make when you are really trying to solve a problem. MindFitness quiets the mind.

♦ Increased happiness and a sense of well-being. It feels good when your alpha levels go up.

♦ Decreased depression. As your alpha sense of calmness and well-being increases, your beta-based depression naturally wanes.

♦ Increased ability to break bad habits. Many people drink, take drugs, and overeat to create a feeling they don't have or to numb a feeling they don't want. When you learn how to change your moods by changing your brain waves, you no longer need mind-altering substances.

At Canyon Ranch we take pride in being open to new techniques and aware of the latest technology, and we believe that MindFitness is one of the most exciting new fitness tools to come along in a great while. Developed more than 15 years ago by Dr. James Hardt at Carnegie Mellon University and the University of California at San Francisco, MindFitness has only recently been moved out of the lab and into the public eye. Canyon Ranch is the first public place where the service is offered.

Virtually everyone who has experienced MindFitness says that it's exhilarating, provocative, and powerful and that its effects are long lasting. No one says that it's easy or something you master overnight. MindFitness training calls for four hours a day for five consecutive days.

THE LAST WORD

As strange as it may seem, many overstressed people find relaxing to be very unrelaxing indeed. For instance, meditation and progressive relaxation make some people anxious. Like all new behaviors, relaxation must be learned and practiced. It's possible that a certain technique isn't right for you—meditation isn't for everyone, for instance, and neither is yoga or progressive relaxation—but you won't know that unless you give it a fair try. If relaxation feels strange, it may be because you're so used to being tense, you feel odd once that the tension is gone. Keep at it.

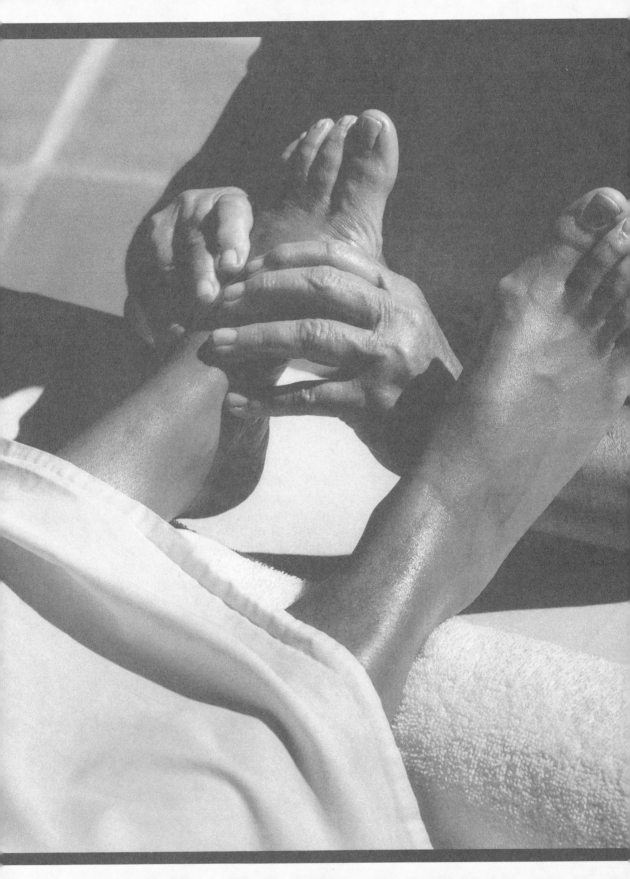

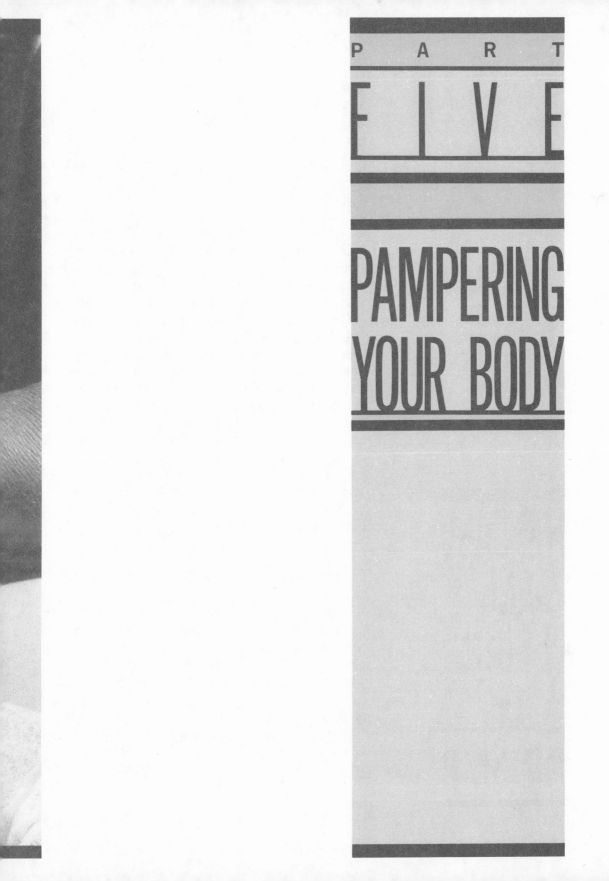

PAMPERING YOUR BODY

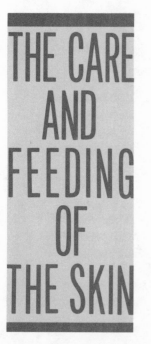

18

THE CARE AND FEEDING OF THE SKIN

I t's not hard to figure out who runs the skin care department at Canyon Ranch. She's the one with the parasol. Leah Kovitz, who's been on the staff of the Ranch since the beginning, practices what she preaches. What she preaches is not vanity, although she's realistic enough to know that people care very much about how they look. No, like everyone else here, Leah preaches the gospel of prevention.

If you're making a list of the ten most important elements of good health, skin care would not be as high up as lowering cholesterol or controlling obesity, but it, along with the other subjects in this section of the book, is still an essential part of the "wellness package." Caring for your skin has both direct and indirect benefits: it makes your skin look and feel better right away; and it balances a lot of hard work with some restorative pampering. After a hard day of avoiding brownies and showing the rowing machine who's boss it's vitally important to pamper yourself at least a little.

How the Skin Ages

Your skin, all 25 square feet and roughly 20 pounds of it, is made up largely of collagen, which provides the skin's framework; elastin, which gives it resiliency; and melanin, which gives it protective coloration. As the years pass and nature takes its course, everyone produces less collagen and elastin, which makes the skin sag and crease. Melanin starts to collect in clumps, which lead to "liver spots" and other blemishes. The outer layer of your skin becomes thinner too, and cell turnover slows down, so that dead skin cells begin to build up on the surface of the skin.

Those changes in the skin are perfectly natural, but serious skin damage has very little to do with Mother Nature. It has everything to do with man- and woman-made hazards, such as unnecessary exposure to the sun, smoking, air pollution, bad diet, and lack of care.

WHAT CAN HELP

Of course, everyone's skin is unique, with a different genetic makeup, and everyone's skin reacts differently to the elements. When it comes to the skin, geography is often destiny: New Yorkers and other easterners have harsh winters, which tend to dilate the capillaries under the skin; most Californians get too much sun; here in the Southwest our skin is starved for moisture. However, no matter where you live or how you spend your time or what your ethnic background is, your skin can benefit from protection and nourishment. Here's how those two general areas break down.

STAY OUT OF THE SUN

Public Skin Enemy #1 is the sun, and for good reason. Skin cancers account for more than half of all malignancies in the United States every year, and 90 percent of all skin cancers result from sun exposure. Common skin cancers affect about 500,000 Americans a year. In 25 years that number could be doubled. Even if you're unlikely to develop skin cancer (fair-skinned people run the highest risk), the sun doesn't do you any favors; at the very least it dries out the skin, causing lines and wrinkles.

There's no way around the fact that the days of oiling up our bodies and baking in the sun all day are gone, or at least they should be. The best thing you can do for your skin is to avoid direct exposure to the sun completely. The next best thing is to wear a good sunscreen, which means learning to play the SPF game. All sunscreens are labeled with an SPF (Sun Protection Factor) number, which refers to the length of time that a person may be in the sun unprotected without burning. A sunscreen rated SPF 15, for example, will let you stay in the sun 15 times as long as usual before you burn. Hypothetically at least, wearing SPF 30 means you can be outside 30 times as long.

It stands to reason that the higher your sunscreen's SPF is, the more protection you'll get from it, and naturally there is a temptation to buy products with a higher number because it makes you think you're getting more value for your money. At the moment, however, the subject of SPF numbers is subject to some debate. Officially the FDA recognizes Sun Protection Factors from 2 to 15 only, yet companies are introducing products that go as high as SPF 39, for what they call "maximum sun protection." The consensus seems to be that opting for numbers in the stratosphere doesn't do any harm, and some experts say that using a higher than necessary number may make up for the fact that people don't apply enough sunscreen to begin with or reapply it often enough.

A sunscreen is effective only if you put enough of it on and keep it on. Going for a swim and then drying yourself off with a towel doesn't leave you with much protection, even if the SPF of the sunscreen you originally applied is 102. Choose one that's waterproof and apply it often.

Keep in mind that there's no such thing as sunblock except a thick, opaque substance, such as zinc oxide—or a shirt. Remember too that the beach is only the most obvious place where you get too much sun. There are plenty of other times when a sunscreen is called for; you can get just as burned when you're gardening, sitting in the right field bleachers, and even strolling along the city streets.

And by the way, basking in a tanning machine is not a safe alternative to bathing in the sun. (If The American Academy of Dermatology had its way, there would be warnings printed on tanning machines.) Because they use intense ultraviolet light exposure, which duplicates the acute and chronic effects of sunlight, machines are perfectly capable of causing skin to age, degenerate, and even develop cancer. What's more, they do their work faster than the sun—15 minutes in a machine is the rough equivalent of an hour in the sun—and because they're private, they encourage you to expose parts of your body that have never seen the sun.

QUIT SMOKING

Smoking slows the circulation of blood to your skin, it releases clouds of dry, dirty smoke into your face, and it makes you purse your lips and squint on a regular basis. As you can imagine, none of these conditions is good for the skin; in fact, a 45-year-old heavy smoker may have skin that looks as many as ten years older. For this and many other reasons, you have to quit smoking. (See Chapter 23.)

TRY THE "GREAT SKIN" DIET

Sorry, there is no such thing, at least not specifically, as a great-skin diet. The best thing for your skin is a sensible diet, one that is high in complex carbohydrates and fiber (especially cereals and other grains, fresh fruits, and fresh vegetables) and low in fat. Be sure you get four to six ounces of protein a day; one of the effects of a protein deficiency is unhealthy looking skin. Drinking lots of water is good for every kind of skin; six to eight cups a day can make a big difference in your appearance. Don't believe the ads you see for creams or lotions that add vitamins, minerals, and other nutritional supplements made "especially for the skin." If your diet is missing something, add a daily multivitamin/mineral supplement; topical preparations are not effective.

THE ACNE-CHOCOLATE CONNECTION

We don't recommend the Chocolate Diet, but we do want to set the record straight: despite the clichés, acne is much more likely to be caused by hormones and heredity than by candy bars or cola. Even a high-fat diet doesn't necessarily lead to skin break-outs. There may be a coincidental relationship, though, since people tend to eat chocolate when they're depressed, under stress, or otherwise emotionally upset, and those emotions, which often have hormonal causes, can lead to bad skin. The same thing that makes your face break out makes you crave chocolate.

GET MOVING

Any kind of exercise is good for the skin, but aerobic exercise, which is particularly good for your circulation and digestion, is best. See Chapter 7 for the specifics.

WATCH OUT FOR HEAT

As you'll see in Chapter 19, at the Ranch we're big fans of steam, saunas, and whirlpool baths. We recommend them very highly for easing tired, achy muscles and for general relaxation. We also encourage people who are feeling the effects of nicotine, alcohol, caffeine, or sugar withdrawal to "sweat it out." Unfortunately, however, for some people, particularly those with fair or sensitive skin, these therapies are not quite so beneficial to the skin as they are to the soul.

If you have oily skin, spending time in the sauna or steam room may make your face, chest, or back break out; all that heat stimulates the sebaceous oil glands. If your skin is on the dry side, a sauna can cause you to become drier still, since you can ill afford to lose oils. And if you have sensitive skin or broken capillaries, heating up your face can make the condition worse. If you can't resist the therapeutic attractions of heat—and most people can't—here are a few precautions you should take:

♦ For oily skin: Clean your face thoroughly before you go in, removing all traces of makeup. Wash again soon after you come out.

♦ For dry skin: Moisturize your face before you go in and soon after you get out. That will trap what little moisture there is on your skin.

◆ For broken capillaries: Keep your face cool by pressing a cold, wet washcloth against your skin. Even with the cool cloth don't stay in the sauna or steam for more than a few minutes, ten at the most. Don't rub your skin afterward.

Whirlpool baths are both good and bad for the skin: on the one hand they massage deep into the tissues, which helps circulation, which in turn helps the skin; on the other hand the heat of the whirlpool robs the skin of moisture. Before you get into a whirlpool put moisturizer on your face and neck.

DO SOMETHING ABOUT STRESS

Stress is bad for just about everything, including the skin. Exercise can help here, but learning to relax and manage stress is better. See Chapter 17 for more about stress management techniques.

ESTABLISH A SKIN CARE REGIMEN

The words "skin care regimen" are downright chilling to some people. They summon up an image of spending hours in front of the bathroom mirror every day, hoping no one will see them with that "goop" on their faces. You couldn't be more wrong. Taking care of your skin is not a full-time job; in only a few minutes a day you can do everything you need to have healthy looking skin. If you don't believe that's all there is to it, keep reading.

THE THREE BASIC STEPS TO HEALTHY SKIN

1   Every night. Clean and moisturize your face, using a cleanser that's right for your skin type and the softest cloth you can find. At the Ranch we use a product called a Skin Shammy, but a diaper will work beautifully. Follow the cleansing with a toner, which should be applied with a cotton ball. (Toner pH-balances the skin and removes any residue of the cleanser.) Finally, moisturize your skin. If you have dry skin, that means applying night cream (a heavy moisturizer) and eye cream. For oily skin you'll need a regular moisturizer and eye cream. Do this as early in the evening as possible; otherwise some of the moisturizer will end up on your pillow, not your face. Try to get in the habit of cleaning your face as soon as you get home in the evening.
2   Every morning. Rinse your face with water and apply a day moisturizer. Apply makeup if you like.
3   Once a week. Use a facial masque for your skin type.
      For dry skin mix 1 egg yolk, 3 tablespoons sesame oil, 3 tablespoons safflower oil, and 1 tablespoon corn oil. Stir in 1 tablespoon cider

vinegar and add 2 drops of fragrance if you like. Apply the mixture over your entire face (or any part of your body that needs special attention) and let it stay there for about 30 minutes. Rinse it off with cold water and apply a moisturizer.

For normal to oily skin mix 2 teaspoons of plain yogurt, ½ teaspoon of fresh lemon juice, and ½ teaspoon of honey. Apply the mixture to your face and neck and let it stay there for about 20 minutes. Clean off the mask with warm water and a soft cloth and apply a moisturizer.

THE RIGHT STUFF

Remember the last time you decided to make yourself over? You probably marched to the cosmetics counter of your city's finest department store and had a chat with the "skin consultant" behind the counter. You explained what you were looking for, asking her advice about what would be best for your kind of skin. Five or ten minutes later you walked away with your package, filled with the line of products she recommended—moisturizer, toner, cleanser, and so on—and eager to go home and take a look at the new you. What you probably don't realize is that virtually every customer this expert speaks to, regardless of skin type, walks away with the same package. Chances are the woman behind the counter doesn't have any idea what she's talking about.

When it comes to finding products that work for your skin, it's a jungle out there, and unfortunately the only way you can make it through the jungle is by finding your own way. Asking dermatologists for advice can be frustrating; understandably enough, they're a lot more interested in, and informed about, diseases of the skin than they are about warding off dry patches and crow's feet. For every two doctors who tell a patient that it's okay to wash her face with soap there is at least one woman who's skin is dry and tight.

You have to experiment until you find a product line you like. Be sure that the line makes cleanser, toner, moisturizer, and eye cream, since it's a good idea not to mix. If you use a toner from one company and a moisturizer from another, the chemicals may clash and have a negative effect on your skin. Companies design their products to work together.

It's also good to change brands every once in a while. If you use the same product for too long—longer than a couple of years—your body may become "immune" to its healing properties. At the Ranch Leah saves our guests the trouble of switching to another brand; she changes the formula of her products every two years.

A SKIN CARE GLOSSARY

When you go shopping, it's important to understand the language of labels. Here are some of the words you'll come across most often:

♦ Hypoallergenic. This means that a product is unlikely to sensitize skin or cause an allergic reaction. Most cosmetics are hypoallergenic.

♦ Non-comedogenic. This means that the product doesn't cause white-heads or blackheads on rabbits' ears, which resemble human skin.

♦ Dermatologist-tested. Just what it sounds like—tested by the doctors themselves.

♦ Fragrance-free. This product has no fragrance whatsoever, as opposed to "unscented," which may contain a scent that masks another scent.

♦ Hypoacnegenic. This means that the product is unlikely to cause acne.

SKIN CARE FOR JOCKS

Makeup and exercise are not a good combination for the skin, especially if you work up a halfway decent sweat while you're at it. When you exercise, your metabolism speeds up, producing more than the usual amount of oil. If your skin is clean, the oil can be released, but if your pores are clogged with makeup, oil can build up. Skin that is-hot, wet, and irritable is particularly sensitive to any foreign substances; sunscreens, tinted moisturizers, and anything that contains fragrance may irritate a hot, perspiring face. If you have sensitive skin, you should make every effort to remove all traces of makeup before you exercise.

Even if you're one of the lucky ones with not-so-sensitive skin, you're better off without makeup when you work out, but if the natural look is unthinkable, keep in mind that a water-based foundation is better for a perspiring face than an oil-based product. Better yet, try to get away with tinted moisturizer or a little loose powder. If you need some roses in your cheeks in addition to the ones you get from your push-ups or your morning jog, opt for gel, which stains the skin instead of clogging it up.

SKIN CARE'S THREE BIGGEST LIES

There are many misconceptions about skin care, but three stand out:

1   Moisturizers make your skin moist. No, they don't, despite the name. Water makes your skin moist, and moisturizer traps the water on your skin. That's why we suggest applying moisturizer to a damp face and spritzing yourself with water a few times a day. Another thing moisturizers don't do is permanently change the composition of your

skin, so the ad copy explaining how and why collagen changes skin texture are exaggerations, to put it mildly. The skin is nourished not from the outside in but from the inside out. If your skin is dry, moisturizer will probably make you look and feel better, but it will have no permanent effect.

2   There are creams that keep you from aging. Ever since Cleopatra people have wanted younger-looking skin. In her day Cleopatra probably had sales clerks telling her that asp placenta would keep her looking great forever. Today we have "anti-aging creams," fortified with such ingredients as collagen, placenta, and special skin vitamins and minerals, and so far Americans have spent about $400 million on them. The money may not be entirely wasted, since many of the creams improve the appearance of the skin. What they do not do, however, is change the skin or reverse the aging process; in fact, no non-prescription skin care product can legally claim to alter the structure of the skin. To keep your skin looking young, eat right, get regular exercise, don't smoke, stay out of the sun, and think beautiful thoughts.

3   You can speed up "cell turnover." Actually this isn't officially a lie; it's more of a half-truth. As a person gets older, the process of sloughing off old skin and replacing it with new takes longer. There are products that claim to increase the cell turnover speed, and some of them do just that. What they are unlikely to say in their claims is that some of the chemicals that encourage the cells to turn over may damage the new skin. After all, burn victims have increased "cell turnover" too.

ALL ABOUT FACIALS

How many people do you know who have to schedule their facials at the end of the day, when they know that they won't have to see anybody (or be seen) for at least 12 hours? That's how long it takes for their skin to look normal after it's been steamed and scrubbed to within an inch of its life.

About one out of five people have what is normally thought of as "sensitive skin" on their faces: very dry, very fair, and often with broken capillaries. They burn easily and practically never tan, and most of them absolutely hate facials. It's easy to understand why, since they usually emerge from the salon looking as if they've gone a few rounds. Many salons go through the same ritual for all their customers, regardless of skin type. Sensitive skin gets peeled and steamed; oily skin gets coated with grease.

Steaming the face stimulates the skin, causing it to lose oil and very possibly creating broken capillaries. It's definitely not recommended for people with sensitive skin; in fact, the only time steam is really necessary is to soften the skin as part of an in-depth facial for somebody who has acne or other impurities around the T-zone (forehead, nose, and chin). Scrubbing and peeling are also inadvisable for the sensitive-skinned.

At the Ranch we believe that facials should make you look and feel wonderful, and we also feel that the best tool to use on the face is the hand. We'll match our massages against machines any day.

THE PROPER WAY TO DEEP-CLEAN YOUR FACE

Some people just aren't happy unless they've had at least a little steam on their faces. If you're one of them, try this relatively gentle deep-cleaning method.

Tie your hair back and clean your face. If you have dry or normal skin, apply a light moisturizer. Fill a sink or large pot with very hot water and lean over the water for five minutes. Tissue off the moisturizer and apply a mask to cool your skin and close the pores. (If your skin is dry or sensitive, choose a creamy mask. For normal skin the best choice is a gel. If you have oily skin, try clay or mud.) Even if you have the sturdiest skin imaginable, it's not a good idea to do this more than three times a week.

THE REST OF YOU

It's the skin on our faces we worry about most, for good reason; after all, it's out there almost all the time, exposed to sun and wind and dirt and anything else the world cares to throw at it. It's no surprise that the skin on the body ages much more slowly than the skin on our faces. However, that does not mean that we should ignore it. Body skin can benefit from a little tender loving care too.

Here are a few tips:

♦ Showers are better for the skin than baths; baths can be very dehydrating to the skin. Take baths only once or twice a week. For best results throw in some herbs, Epsom salts, or (especially in wintertime) some fragrant oil.

♦ Use a loofah in the shower; it improves your circulation while it cleans, and it sloughs off dead skin. Use a loofah just like a sponge: put soap on it and scrub gently.

♦ To keep your skin moist after a bath or shower blot your body almost dry with a towel and apply moisturizer or body lotion over the water drops that remain. The water, nature's moisturizer, is trapped under the lotion.

♦ Body massage is wonderful for the skin. Almost any kind of massage is good, but Swedish is the overall favorite.

It's a real struggle to keep the skin on your hands smooth and moist. So many things conspire to dry them out, among them soap and water, the elements, and excessive paper-shuffling. Wash your hands with a mild, superfatted soap and be sure to rinse them thoroughly. Pat them almost dry and apply hand cream. (If you can't stand the greasy feeling on the palms of your hands, wipe it off.) If you cream your hands only once in a while, remember that the best time for hand cream is at night, when the hands are clean and not likely to be soaked in water for a while. If your hands have taken a special beating, smear them with petroleum jelly before you go to bed and wear a pair of cotton gloves. Other tips for hand care: soak your nails in lukewarm water to replenish moisture; use a polish remover without acetone; try a facial mask on your hands every so often; and when you're applying sunscreen, don't forget to dab a little on your hands.

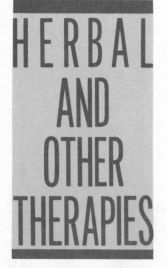

HERBAL AND OTHER THERAPIES

19

44"I went through terrible withdrawal pains," the woman was saying to her spellbound audience. "It started with headaches and stomach cramps, and then I was burning up with fever. I became dizzy and disoriented, too, and I couldn't sleep. There were times when I really thought I was going to die. Eventually I had to check into a hospital until I could kick the habit completely." The rapt listeners the woman was addressing were the participants in the Canyon Ranch "Managing Your Food Habits" program. The grisly scene she described was giving up sugar.

Our bodies are virtual chemistry labs. Every day we synthesize chemicals at an extraordinary rate, coping with smog, fumes, alcohol, coffee, smoke, over-the-counter and prescription drugs, and the various additives in our food. The liver, bowel, bladder, and kidneys work overtime to remove the poisons, as do the respiratory system and the skin, but even so, we sometimes build up a level of toxicity that our bodies just can't handle. Our systems were designed thousands of years ago, and not for cigarettes, dry martinis, refined sugar, or eight cups of coffee a day. Neanderthal man did not have to cope with chocolate eclairs and toxic waste.

The strange thing is, our bodies become accustomed to many of these poisons, which is why withdrawal from them can be so grim. The body is a creature of habit, and when it doesn't get what it has come to expect, it starts to look for it, to call the substance "out of storage" in the bloodstream. A biological change actually takes place, and although the change is for the better, often it makes us feel a lot worse before we get better. When the woman we described above didn't get her "fix" of sugar, her body rebelled. That's what withdrawal is and why you're inclined to feel so rotten when you quit smoking or eliminate drugs, alcohol, caffeine, and sugar from your system.

DETOX THERAPIES

Detoxification is a scary-sounding word, but it's an appropriate description of what happens when you begin to get rid of the various poisons in your body. Because it's not often a very pleasant process, the more quickly it is accomplished, the better off you are. One of the best ways to speed things up is to stimulate the body's eliminative abilities, and one of the best ways to do that is to sweat it out. At the Ranch we suggest drinking a couple of quarts of water a day (a good habit to get into anyway) and lots of vigorous exercise. We also tell our guests to spend time in the steam room, sauna, and whirlpool baths and to try the herbal wraps and baths, ideally a treatment on three consecutive days.

These therapies are by no means new. The combination of heat (wet or dry), water (hot or cold), and herbs has been with us for centuries. Long before boils were lanced, for instance, they were coated with clay to "draw out the poisons," and people were routinely swathed in layers of blankets until their fevers broke. They're also not untested; the reason they're still around is that they work. "Health practices that don't work usually disappear," says Deborah Morris, the resident expert on herbal healing. "Notice how bloodletting and leeching have fallen into disfavor."

Virtually everyone can benefit from these therapies, and not just for detoxification. They also increase circulation, promote relaxation, and, as long as you don't abuse them, improve the quality of your skin. They're a wonderful tool for stress management, if only because they give you some "down" time to let the mind and body connect. People react in different ways to the various treatments, which is why we encourage a kind of Chinese menu approach—one from column A, one from column B—to choosing the therapy that's right for you. For best results, try them all.

STEAM, SAUNAS, AND JACUZZIS

Remember those scenes from early comedies showing the fat man who goes into a steam cabinet and (after being left alone for hours) comes out reduced to a fraction of his original size? Lies, all lies. Spending time in steam rooms, saunas, and jacuzzis won't make you lose weight. It's true that your heart beats faster and you begin to sweat, but no actual aerobic activity is involved. Your heart isn't sending more oxygen to your muscles, so you don't burn fat. (You do lose water and salt, though, which is why the scale may register weight loss right after a session in the sauna. That weight is gained back as soon as you drink a glass of water.) As a weight loss method these therapies work about as well as watching a movie.

They're wonderful for other things, though, including detoxification, relaxation, and easing soreness in the muscles. They can be especially refreshing after you've been exercising strenuously, and some people use them to warm up before class too.

All the therapies—steam, sauna, inhalation therapy, and whirlpool baths—are equally effective; the one that works best for you is the one you enjoy the most. A sauna uses dry heat, and it tends to work more deeply because it takes longer to raise your core temperature. It also tends to make people a little claustrophobic if they are so inclined. Steam rooms give off moist heat, which works a little more quickly to open pores and speed up circulation. Jacuzzis are more sociable, and they're easier on the hair and facial skin. Inhalation rooms (especially kind to clogged sinuses) may use either wet or dry heat, depending on the weather. Here in Tucson ours are wet to counter the effects of our dry climate.

If you're pregnant, if you have phlebitis, or if you have a skin rash, you should stay away from saunas, steam, and jacuzzis. If you have hypertension or heart disease, you should get your doctor's permission before you take the plunge. Even ten minutes in a sauna or steam room can make your heart beat twice as fast as usual; that kind of stress may be too much for a weak heart. If none of these things apply, start experimenting. Here are some tips to keep in mind:

♦ Don't stay in any of the treatments for too long. A 15-minute session is about right.

♦ If your skin is sensitive (very dry or very fair) or if you have broken capillaries on your face, proceed with caution. Don't stay in for more than eight to ten minutes and protect your face with a cold wet wash cloth.

♦ The temperature should be no higher than 120 degrees. Check the thermostat. If there is no thermostat, don't use the room.

♦ It's best to remove all of your clothes, but always lie or sit on a towel. Take off your jewelry too; it can burn you.

♦ Don't go in right after eating a meal. Wait for at least an hour.

♦ Replace the oils and fluids you lost as soon as you come out. Have a glass of water and moisturize your skin with lotion or oil.

♦ If you have a cold, put some Tiger Balm under each nostril.

♦ For a nice heat treatment for your hair, apply a conditioner and wear a shower cap.

HERBAL WRAPS AND BATHS

In the olden days people's homes had a distinctive smell: bread baking in the oven, soup on the top of the stove, herbs drying in the window, fresh flowers in the living room, lavender in the baby's room to keep it germ-free, or all of the above. The prevailing thought then was that virtually everything that grows—pollen, seeds, mud, roots, flowers, and herbs—has some medicinal use. At the Ranch we believe that too, and one of the most useful purposes we can imagine for herbs are wraps and baths.

The herbal wrap room may well be the most soothing, relaxing place at Canyon Ranch. The lights are dim, the music is soft, and the herbal tea is plentiful. No one speaks above a whisper, and there's a lovely exotic scent in the air. The only trouble is that most of the people in the room can't move, because they're trapped under several layers of hot, herb-soaked sheets. The strange thing is, they like it!

AROMATHERAPY

It probably won't come as a great surprise to you to learn that we are affected by smell. Scent has always been used therapeutically: to relax, to stimulate, to heal, even to relieve pain. Only recently, however, have we begun to make a study of what is being called aromatherapy and to discover that it may have an effect on our heart rate, blood pressure, and hormones. Aromatherapy has been used to treat everything from respiratory distress to chronic depression. Sometimes essential oils are introduced through inhalation; other times they are applied topically, as they are in our dry wraps; and occasionally herbal essences are placed under the tongue and taken internally.

Various smells affect the way we feel and how we think, partly because we have scent memories: pine needles invoke thoughts of Christmas past, Chanel No. 5 means Mom, lilac bushes remind you of your friend's backyard, and every time you get a whiff of chlorine, you think about afternoons in junior high. Some smells make us feel invigorated; others we find relaxing. Some make us happy, some sad. Since everyone reacts differently to different smells, you have to experiment with various herbs and flower essences to discover which ones you enjoy and which ones bring about the healing process you're looking for. The bad news is that the experiments may take some time; the good news is that it will be time very pleasantly spent.

One of the pleasantest (and most therapeutic) imaginable ways to spend 30 minutes is soaking in a fragrant bath. Fill a tub with comfortably warm water and add ten drops of herb-essence oil. Rub your skin with a little of the oil, and step into the tub.

Herbal wraps are incredibly soothing and rejuvenating, but they are not to everyone's taste, at least not right away. Enid Zuckerman herself used to feel trapped by the wraps; she had to try it a dozen times before she could stay wrapped up for a full half hour without being at least a little anxious. Even dyed-in-the-wool claustrophobics like Enid can learn to love the wraps, provided the therapist knows what he or she is doing (and doesn't disappear out of easy reach) and as long as you wrap only as much of your body as you can stand. Enid started by leaving her feet and arms out; then it was just her arms; now she opts for a total wrap.

Some herbal wraps are dry; we call ours aromatherapy wraps. In this variation an aromatic formula is rubbed and placed strategically on your skin. Then you are wrapped in several layers of dry cloths, and a small amount of heat is introduced by means of an electric blanket. In addition to promoting detoxification and relaxation dry wraps relieve poor circulation, congestion, indigestion, and PMS.

Many folks who never develop a fondness for wraps swear by herbal baths. Most of the time this is just a matter of personal taste, but in a few special cases baths really are better than wraps. Because the concentration of the herbal mixture is greater in the bath than in the wraps and because the bath lets you breathe the fumes, baths are particularly effective in the treatment of deep congestion, upper respiratory infections, asthma, and sinus infections. The baths are also wonderful tension-reducers.

An Herbal Primer

Basil aids digestion; chamomile calms you down and helps clear up acne; eucalyptus acts as a stimulant and opens the sinuses; lavender is an effective antiseptic; lemon is a diuretic, good for skin tone; peppermint is a stimulant, helpful for fatigue; and rose is a cleanser and good for getting rid of headaches. There are no engraved-in-stone rules, no specific formulas for healing, when it comes to herbal therapy; in fact, the recipe for the herb mixture we use in the wrap room at the Ranch changes every couple of months. Herbs have specific identifiable properties, often more than one. Ours is a mixture of native southwestern herbs containing at least one herb from each of three categories: muscle relaxants, nervines (for the nervous system), and diaphoritics (herbs that raise body temperature and stimulate detoxification). We also include an herb that re-establishes the pH balance of the skin.

There is plenty of room for creativity and experimentation, and we encourage you to try different combinations yourself. Visit your health food store or send away for mail-order catalogs. Talk to people about what has worked well for them. This brief list should help you get started.

♦ Astringents: vinegar, sage, comfrey, nettle, chamomile, sandalwood, rosemary, mint, rose, and lavender.

♦ Antiseptics: chamomile, mint, lavender, thyme, eucalyptus, sandalwood, and rosemary.

♦ Skin tonics: lavender, rosemary, thyme, lemon, mint, and nettle.

♦ Cleansers: elder, fennel, lovage, lavender, yarrow, rose.

♦ Skin soothers: oatmeal, cornmeal, cider vinegar, dandelion, elder, lemon, calendula, comfrey, nettle.

♦ Skin softeners: elder, fennel, rose, linden.

♦ Deodorizers: lovage and sage.

♦ Muscle relaxers: marjoram, vinegar, salt, chamomile, rose, lemon, mint, yarrow, and lavender.

♦ Muscle stimulants: eucalyptus and wintergreen.

♦ Moisturizers: orange blossom, chamomile, and rose.

♦ Healers: mint, chamomile, elder, linden, and rosemary.

♦ Circulation stimulants: thyme, lavender, peppermint, rosemary, and pine.

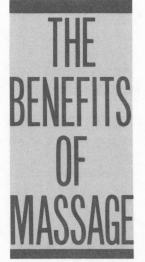

20

THE
BENEFITS
OF
MASSAGE

"I have a massage every night. Sometimes I think it's the only thing that keeps me going," said one man as he set off on the four-mile walk at seven o'clock one morning. Others were quick to agree. "I walked four miles, took two aerobics classes, went to two stretch classes, and took a tennis lesson yesterday," a woman offered. "If I hadn't had a massage last night, I'm sure I couldn't have gotten out of bed this morning." What these guests (and practically everyone else who comes to the Ranch) have discovered are the healing properties of touch.

Long before there was our Positive Power class there was massage. One theory has it that it started with Hippocrates, whose brother was a massage therapist. Over the years it's gone in and out of fashion—out in the Middle Ages, back in during the Renaissance. In this country there was a massage boom after World War II and another one in the sixties, and while it still does not enjoy the stature in the United States that it has in Europe, it appears to be here to stay.

The bad news is that massage doesn't make you lose weight, get rid of cellulite, or make lines and wrinkles disappear. The good news is that it does just about everything else. The benefits of massage are physical, psychological, even spiritual.

PHYSICAL BENEFITS

Our bodies contain about 22 miles of arteries and veins, which are kept active by the contraction and relaxation of the muscles. If any part of that system becomes choked (through a great deal of exercise or stress, for instance) chemical deposits, sometimes detected as "knots," form in the body. The primary function of massage is to break up these crystalline formations so that they can be carried out of the system. In addition to aiding circulation and speeding detoxification massage helps to keep muscles in tone, reduce swelling and inflammation, improve digestion, and keep the body supple. It's even good for the skin. Athletes swear by massage, relying on it as part of their physical therapy programs. Many arthritis and osteoporosis sufferers have discovered its joys as well. There is no one who cannot derive a physical benefit from some sort of massage.

PSYCHOLOGICAL BENEFITS

Massage is good for the head too. One of the favorite maxims of fitness director Karma Kientzler is, "If you don't get ten hugs a day, you're not healthy." She doesn't mean that literally, of course (seven or eight hugs may be plenty), but Karma does believe, as we all do, that touching is essential to well-being. Studies have shown that infants and children who are picked up and held often are much healthier than those who aren't. Massage can teach as well as nurture, by making you more aware of your body. For instance, post-surgical patients and accident victims who are finding it difficult to acknowledge an injured body part may be helped by massage. Massage makes almost everyone more sensitive to touch and more open to trusting others.

MENTAL/SPIRITUAL BENEFITS

Massage nourishes the mind and the spirit too, giving you time to relax, clear your head, and think beautiful thoughts. Extremely calming to the sympathetic nervous system, massage may also affect the brain waves, making it easier to move into the creative alpha state. (For more about brain waves see Chapter 17.) If you're feeling angry, anxious, or unhappy, massage can put you back on an even keel.

THE BEST MASSAGE

At a little before seven o'clock one evening the woman was reading a magazine in the spa building and waiting for her massage. She had been at the Ranch for about ten days and had tried several kinds of massage: Swedish, shiatsu, reflexology, even cranial. Even though she had never had a massage before coming to the Ranch, she was starting to feel like an old hand at it.

When she heard her name called, she followed the spa attendant to the massage therapy room. The massage therapist introduced himself and then left the room for a moment so that she could remove her robe and lie on the table under the sheet. When he returned, he began massaging her head, working in silence for a couple of minutes. "Have you ever had a massage before?" he asked, moving to her shoulders.

"Sure," the woman responded. "I've had four or five."

Another few minutes passed, and the therapist, who had reached her back, asked, "Do you enjoy massage?"

"Yes, I do," she replied. "I'm new at it, but I'm really starting to like it."

Five minutes went by, and he spoke again. "Let me take a wild guess," he said. "Is this the first time you've been worked on by a man?"

The woman burst out laughing. "What gave me away?" she inquired. "Do I seem tense?"

"A little," he replied, "but that's okay. I've never actually worked on an ironing board before!"

Of course, the massage therapist was right. It was the woman's first time with a male therapist, and she was self-conscious and nervous. She thought she could be nonchalant about it, but the body can't tell a lie.

One of the reasons the woman had decided to make her appointment with a male therapist that evening was that she had heard some of the women talking about how men give better massages than women. "No way," another group responded. "Sometimes they're stronger than women, but they're definitely not better." This led into one of the most hotly debated subjects at the Ranch: Who gives the best massage?

The answer is simple: the best massage is not the one given by a woman or a man, not the one that's gentle or much more firm but the one that makes you feel best. What you like may depend on many things: the type of massage, the technique and style of the individual therapist, and the rapport you have with the therapist. To make the most of a massage, you have to relax, and the only way you can do that is to trust the therapist. You have to be confident that he or she won't hurt you or make you uncomfortable in any way.

Although the strokes may be the same and the therapists equally qualified, every massage you have will be different, not just because of the therapist but also because of the attitude you bring to the experience. The more relaxed you are during a massage, the more you'll get out of it. If you have a hard time relaxing and "giving in" to a massage, prepare yourself for it by having an herbal wrap first or spending a few minutes in the sauna, steam room, or jacuzzi. If you start to tense up on the table, take deep, cleansing breaths. Visualize yourself in a relaxed state. It sounds strange, but it's true: getting a massage takes practice.

Don't be afraid to tell the therapist what you want. All therapists have a preferred technique, but they'll be glad to adapt it a bit to suit your preference—to work a little lighter or a little deeper or to avoid a very sensitive spot, for instance. Massage is not supposed to hurt, but only you can decide where to draw the line; if the therapist is hurting you, say so. A massage that makes you uncomfortable is not likely to do your body or your psyche much good.

If one of the things about massage that makes you uncomfortable is taking off all of your clothes in front of strangers, men or women, you're not alone. You're also not out of luck. You can get the enjoyment of massage while remaining fully clothed if you try shiatsu, reflexology, cranial massage, and Trager.

DIFFERENT STROKES

It's possible that you're not very interested to know what the massage therapist is doing to you; all you care about is how good it feels. But just in case you're curious—or in case you'd like to try your hand at massage—here's a brief description of the basic massage strokes:

♦ Effleurage. A long stroking motion that calms the nervous system. Usually done at the beginning of a massage.

♦ Petrissage. The deep circular movement of the fingertips or thumbs on a particular muscle or area.

♦ Tapotement. A light, steady tapping that causes a slight vibration.

♦ Kneading. Just what it sounds like. Pretend your body is bread dough.

♦ Friction. Rubbing the surface of the skin with the palms of the hand.

♦ Rocking. Placing your hand on the body and rocking or shaking it gently back and forth.

♦ Feather stroke. A soft, soothing stroke of the fingers.

THE TYPES OF MASSAGE

After Canyon Ranch guests are through debating about who gives the best massage, they can move on to another important question: Which is the best kind? Here are the candidates:

BASIC SWEDISH

Swedish, the most popular and most often requested of all the massages we offer, has become almost a generic term for massage. (According to Patricia Benjamin, the historian of the American Massage Therapy Association, it is only in the United States that it's called Swedish massage, after Pehr Henrik Ling, a Swede who invented what he called "medical gymnastics" in the early 19th century.) The standard Swedish massage involves working through the whole body with effleurage (stroking), and it also includes friction, petrissage, kneading, and tapotement. It's an "all-purpose" massage, since it works all the major muscle groups to increase circulation, relax the whole body, and promote a feeling of well-being. The rhythm of this technique can be slow or vigorous, and the pressure can vary from light to deep according to your wishes and the style of the therapist. It's good before or after strenuous exercise and excellent as part of a program to manage stress.

SPORTS MASSAGE

This is an overall massage too, but it involves deep muscle massage, often around the joints, and resistance stretches. It's particularly recommended for rehabilitating torn or strained muscles.

SHIATSU

The word literally means finger pressure, and many people quite understandably confuse shiatsu with acupressure. Acupressure is Chinese; shiatsu is Japanese. However, both are based on the theory that there are meridians on the body (eight in this case), and that each meridian corresponds to a different organ in the body. When pressure is exerted on these points, energy pathways are stimulated, and contracted muscles are encouraged to relax. Shiatsu also increases blood flow, helps balance the nervous system, and makes you feel energized. No oil is used, so you are welcome to keep your clothes on if you choose.

JIN SHIN JYUTSU

This massage identifies 14 meridians, but unlike shiatsu, jin shin employs a very light, subtle technique, which is based on synchronizing the pulses in two parts of the body. Using a firm yet gentle hold, the therapist works on knots and blocked places in the body, releasing natural pain relievers and rejuvenating the immune system. This method is highly recommended for people who have had injuries, not only because it is gentle but also because it opens up circulation in areas that you may have been "rejecting."

REFLEXOLOGY

Reflexology maintains that the body is divided into ten zones, all of which have a corresponding reflex on the foot. (The hands and ears have the same reflexes.) Using precise pressure on the feet, the reflexologist improves circulation, promotes relaxation, and relieves pain in places that are nowhere near the feet. It's especially good for getting rid of headaches and muscle aches, and it doesn't tickle. You can keep your clothes on if you like, but no shoes and socks are allowed.

CRANIAL MASSAGE

This gentle, quite passive method is especially good for people who have trouble relaxing during massage. Its light, soothing manipulation of the pressure points of the spine, shoulders, neck, and head improves the circulation of cerebral spinal fluid to the entire nervous system. Along the way it can relieve headaches and back problems and help you stop gritting and grinding your teeth.

LYMPHATIC MASSAGE

This slow, light massage of the lymph glands (also called Manual Lymph Drainage) calms the sympathetic nervous system and helps to move toxins out of the system, promoting the normal function of the lymphatic system and enhancing the activity of the immune system. It reduces pain and fluid retention and decreases the discomfort of colds, sinus problems, headaches, and arthritis. It's especially good for relieving the symptoms of lymph edema, but it's not recommended for people suffering from phlebitis.

POLARITY

In some ways polarity is the synthesis of Eastern and Western massage therapies. Developed by an osteopath, it's based on the same meridian principle as shiatsu, and it features light to deep pressure combined with lots of gentle rocking, holding, and stretching of the muscles until the body is in correct alignment.

REIKI

This ancient system of mind-body integration is recommended very highly for people in a diseased state, since it is almost completely passive. Quite simply, the therapist transmits heat from his or her hands to your body. This produces a calming and nurturing effect, which can ease headaches, stomach disorders, even pain from injuries. It's great for relaxation too.

TRAGER

This is another very gentle method, and it's particularly good for people with restricted motion in the joints. Trager involves gentle rocking, stretching, rotation, and compression of the body. It's very helpful in making the body more flexible and relieving tightness in the neck, shoulders, lower back, and chest. No oil is used, so you may stay fully clothed.

How to Give a Great Massage

A couple of times a week, when most of the guests at the Ranch are off listening to a lecture or eating unsalted popcorn in the movie room, a few couples are in one of the gymnasiums giggling. What is causing their giggles is the two-hour massage workshop given by massage therapist Lynn Kerry. Some of the laughter is caused by ticklish participants, but most of it comes because people are having fun. There's some nervous laughter too, as guests learn new skills and find it a little awkward or even a little silly. But after even one session they've learned the basics.

THE RULES

There aren't any rules, or at least there aren't many, and most of them can be bent if not broken. You can give a massage for as long as you like, and you can work on body parts in any order you choose, stroking either toward or away from the heart. You don't have to be strong, and you don't have to be the "nurturing type." If you don't have the time or the inclination to give a full body massage, just working on the head and shoulders or the feet can be quite enough. In fact, as long as you stay away from the throat and from inflamed body parts, almost anything goes. Here are the basics of giving a good massage.

LEARN HOW TO MOVE. In massage *how* you move is much more important than what you do with your hands, because if you don't move right, you don't feel comfortable, and if you don't feel comfortable, you won't give a good massage. Proper posture is critical: stand up straight with your pelvis tucked in and your feet well apart. Always bend from the knees, not the waist, and never let your arms go on a mission by themselves; follow through with your whole body. You'll be tempted to "get your nose into your work," as Lynn Kerry describes it, but remain upright and move your head, elbows, and hips as a unit. Use your body strength when you apply pressure; don't rely just on your hands and fingertips. Alternate detail strokes (petrissage) with general strokes (effleurage); switching from one to the other is soothing to your partner, and it keeps your hands from getting tired. Wear comfortable shoes.

LISTEN TO YOUR PARTNER. Pay attention not just to his words but to his body as well. If you hit a sore or sensitive spot, ease the pressure a bit but keep working—unless the soreness is due to an injury, a sprain, or a bruise. If he resists your touch, move to another spot but return to the sore spot later, gently easing pressure into that area.

PAY ATTENTION TO AMBIENCE. After you've decided to give a massage, take some time to set the scene, with soft lighting (maybe candlelight), incense, relaxing music, and plenty of time. Make sure you're both in the mood for it. If you feel you've been roped into giving a massage, the experience will not be as pleasant as it can and should be. If your partner is cranky or ill-tempered, your efforts will be wasted. Massage should be something you share when you feel good.

GET THE RIGHT EQUIPMENT. The reason massage tables exist is that they are the ideal piece of equipment for the job. A bed is imperfect at best, even if it's a single bed, and while putting a quilt on the floor may be acceptable to the one getting the massage, the person giving it is probably going to end up with a tired back. If you don't have a proper massage table (and you probably don't), cover a sturdy dining room table with a few blankets and give it a try. (You can order a table from Sharper Image, 680 Davis Street, San Francisco, California 94111, 800-344-4444; Pisces Productions, P.O. Box 208, Cotati, California 94928; and Living Earth Craft, 800-358-8292.)

THE TWO MOST COMMON MASSAGE MISTAKES

#1. "Relax." It's amazing how annoying that word can be, especially if it's spoken by someone who is giving a massage. It's amazing too how natural it is to want to say it, when you feel all that tension at your fingertips. Don't do it; it only makes matters worse, and it may even start an argument. If your partner could relax, he would. If she could let her arm go limp and not help you lift it up, she would. And maybe he or she will next time, or the time after that. Meanwhile, communicate your instructions physically, not verbally.

#2. When couples give each other a massage, another natural tendency on the part of the person giving the massage is a desire to "fix" someone—to cure a headache or perform some other medical miracle. It's a big mistake to set goals for a massage. If expectations aren't met, someone ends up feeling cheated, and somebody else feels like a failure instead of having a lovely time sharing an intimate experience. Giving a massage to someone you care for is a generous and loving gesture. Don't weigh it down with unnecessary emotional baggage.

You'll definitely need sheets or towels, as many as are necessary for your partner's comfort. Even if modesty is not an issue, feeling secure is an essential part of the nurturing process. Tuck your partner in gently, uncovering only one body part at a time and then recovering the spot when you're finished with it.

You'll need oil too, a selection of which you'll find at any health food store (rosemary and jasmine are Lynn Kerry's favorites). You can also use baby oil or light vegetable oil. Regular bath oils have too much perfume, and mineral oil is too heavy. Massage creams are fine too, but hand creams won't do; they contain too much water, and they may contain alcohol.

HAVE FUN. If you don't, your partner won't either. Be creative and playful. Don't be afraid to experiment.

THE MAIN EVENT

Here's the outline we follow in our massage workshop. Remember that you don't have to do a full massage; even a partial will be much appreciated.

MASSAGING THE HEAD

1   Ask your partner to lie on his or her back. Center yourself at the head of the table.
2   Hold your partner's head gently. Turn it onto one hand and rub the scalp with your fingertips, using small, deep circles.
3   Find the occipital ridge, the bony ridge at the back of the head that runs from ear to ear. Allowing your partner's head to rest on the table, manipulate the ridge with your fingertips.
4   Spread your thumbs across your partner's forehead and make circles on the jaw with your fingertips.
5   Gently pinch the ears.

MASSAGING THE SHOULDERS

1   Standing directly behind your partner's head, tuck your thumbs in and alternately put your hands under the shoulders and draw up the back of the neck. Keep your own back straight.
2   Bend over, rest your arms on the table, and use your fist to follow the curve of the shoulder and neck.

3   Standing near your partner's wrist, rest your closest hand on that wrist. Then, still with your thumb tucked in, use your other hand to massage the back of the neck and shoulders.

MASSAGING THE ARMS

1   With your arms still resting on the wrist, make long sweeping strokes (effleurage) from your partner's wrist to his shoulder with your other hand.
2   Rest your partner's elbow on the table, hold the wrist, and squeeze toward the elbow with the other hand.
3   Knead his upper arm.

MASSAGING THE HANDS

1   With the person's elbow still on the table, use both your hands to squeeze the whole hand.
2   Then, still supporting the hand, grasp each finger in turn and use it to shake the hand lightly.
3   Pinch and squeeze out each finger.
4   Using your thumbs, massage and spread the palm of the hand with small, hard circles.

MASSAGING THE FRONT OF THE LEGS

1   Standing near the ankle, effleurage the front of the legs with both hands from ankle to hip. Make your body weight work for you; step forward onto your front leg.
2   Make circles around the knee.
3   Knead the thigh.
4   Massage up the legs first with long strokes. Then, using your thumbs, work up the muscled areas of the legs in small strokes.

MASSAGING THE FEET

1   Standing at the end of the table, knead and squeeze the whole foot while pulling it toward you.
2   Pinch and squeeze out each toe.
3   Hold the foot firmly with your outside hand. Make a fist with your inside hand and use your knuckles to work the bottom of the foot.
4   Make circles around your partner's ankle with the fingertips of both hands.
5   Squeeze the heels.

MASSAGING THE BACK OF THE LEGS

1 Ask your partner to turn over onto his stomach slowly. Standing near the ankle, effleurage with both hands from ankle to hip. Use your weight.
2 Sit on the end of the table and rest your partner's ankle on your shoulder. Petrissage and squeeze the calf.
3 Knead the thigh.

RE-MASSAGING THE FEET

1 Stand at the foot of the table. Use both of your hands on both feet at the same time. Make loose fists and use the back of your fingers to stroke the bottoms of the feet.

MASSAGING THE BACK

1 Center yourself at the head of the table.
2 Effleurage the back with both of your hands flat, first down the back (using your weight), then up the sides (with little pressure), then out the shoulders (use your weight again).
3 Petrissage in the upper back triangle, making small circles with your thumbs.
4 Stand near your partner's waist and petrissage in the lower back triangle, using your thumbs and the heels of your hands.
5 With your hands together on your partner's waist, press down, using your weight and ending up with a hand on each side of your partner's waist. Draw your hands back up and press again.
6 Knead your partner's shoulders.
7 Knead your partner's buttocks.
8 Feather stroke your partner's back with your fingertips.
9 Rock your partner gently.
10 Draw the sheet up and feather stroke one last time.

WHERE TO LEARN MORE

The above instructions will enable you to give a perfectly good massage, but after trying it out a few times you may well want to move on to more sophisticated techniques. Other books may help—George Downey's *The Massage Book* is excellent—but you may benefit even more from some hands-on instruction. Massage classes are offered in many different locations. Local colleges and universities, YMCAs, and other community organizations are a good place to start; the Yellow Pages may help. Make sure your teacher has the right credentials for the job. Not every state has licensing procedures for massage therapists, but many do, and so do some cities.

THE TEN-MINUTE SELF-MASSAGE

It's easy to schedule a massage here at the Ranch; we employ more than 55 massage therapists, and we have 25-plus massage rooms available from ten in the morning until nine at night. Unfortunately, however, life out there in the Real World is not so convenient, and it's not always possible to schedule a massage when you think you need one.

For those times there's self-massage. When you feel yourself tightening up, clenching your teeth, or holding your shoulders up somewhere around your ears and you can't stop what you're doing for more than ten minutes, try this.

1   Take three deep, slow breaths.
2   Rotate your shoulders, first backward three times, then forward three times.
3   Using your fingers, massage your temples in a circular motion for 30 seconds. Massage your jaw, concentrating on the hinges. Force yourself to unclench your jaws.
4   Drop your chin onto your chest five times, slowly. Move your right ear to your right shoulder five times. Then switch sides, trying to touch your left ear to your left shoulder five times. Finally, move your chin down to the left and touch your left shoulder. Switch to the right. Go back and forth five times.
5   Cross your arms in front of you and reach around to your shoulders. Using your thumbs and index fingers, knead your trapezius muscle (the one that runs along the top of your back) for about 30 seconds.
6   Place your thumbs just above your eyebrows at the bridge of your nose. Press hard with the flat of your thumb and hold the position for five seconds. Move your thumb along the brow line and repeat, working your way out to the temples.
7   Place your thumbs just *under* your eyebrows at the bridge of your nose. Press hard with the flat of your thumb and hold the position for five seconds. Move the thumb along the brow line and repeat, working your way out to the temples.

21

Quick, what contains a quarter of all the bones in the body and has no business whatsoever wearing high heels? Right, it's your feet, and you probably haven't been paying enough attention to them. When your feet hurt, you hurt all over—back, neck, knees—and you probably don't look so great either; foot problems affect your posture and balance, not to mention the expression on your face. Aching feet also serve as a barometer for the rest of the body. Arthritis, diabetes, heart disease, circulatory problems, and kidney disease may be detected in the feet first.

As you become more active and start moving your body on a regular basis, you should be even more attentive to your feet than ever. In many of our exercise classes we take a few minutes to concentrate on stretching and massaging the feet. It doesn't raise your heart rate, but it does improve your health. When you go through your own workouts, keep in mind that your body doesn't end at the ankles.

ENEMIES OF THE FEET

By the time we reach adulthood, about 70 percent of us have some sort of foot problems. Women suffer four times as many foot ailments as men, something that's easy to understand if you've ever watched a woman walking down the street in stilt-high heels. High fashion isn't the only culprit these days, though. There are a few others.

THE WRONG SHOES

The skin on the soles of your feet is roughly ten times thicker than the skin anywhere else on your

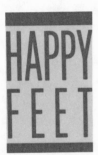

HAPPY FEET

body. Goodness knows we need the padding. The top of the foot isn't so nicely padded, however, which is why corns, blisters, and ingrown toenails develop when ill-fitting shoes rub against the toe. Practically everyone is plagued by corns, blisters, and ingrown toenails at some time or other, but virtually every one of the problems could be avoided with the right shoe. Other injuries, such as stress fractures, bruises, twisted ankles, and even shin splints, can be prevented by wearing shoes with the right kind of support.

Be sure that your shoe fits your activity. Running shoes provide great support for running, but they're wrong for aerobics; if you wear tennis shoes out for a hike, you're asking for trouble.

TIGHT MUSCLES

Sometimes your feet hurt because your muscles, especially the ones in your back, hamstrings, quadriceps, and calves, are too tight or too short. (High-heeled shoes cause calf muscles to contract and tighten.) Strong bones and flexible muscles make your whole system work better. Throw out your high heels or wear them only when you don't plan to do much if any walking or standing. Gentle stretching exercises for the back of the calves help keep you loose.

BAD FORM

If your body is not in proper alignment when you stand and walk and otherwise move around, it can play havoc with your whole body, including your feet. (See Chapter 10 for information on good posture.) If you don't use the right form when you exercise, especially when you run, you can really hurt yourself. Two of the most common flaws are overpronation (feet that turn in too much) and excessive supination (feet that turn out too much). These abnormalities are accentuated when you run or do other strenuous exercise, and both can seriously stress the knee, the least stable joint in the body. Look for shoes that offset your problem, but if a shoe doesn't solve it, you may need an orthotic, an orthopedic device that supports the foot in a neutral, stable position.

OVERDOING IT

If you begin an exercise program too quickly, you may get injured in all sorts of important places. Often the first spot you feel it is your feet. Go easy for a while and then try it again, slowly. If your pain is chronic, you may have chosen the wrong sport or exercise for your body type.

BEING OFF BALANCE

About 90 percent of the population has one leg shorter than the other. Most of the time the discrepancy is small (about a quarter of an inch) and inconsequential, but once in a while it causes a noticeable imbalance, which can lead to pain. Most orthopedists say that a difference of less than a half-inch is not worth correcting. For anything over that you may need an orthotic to restore your balance.

WORKOUTS FOR THE FEET

Any exercise that lengthens and strengthens the muscles, particularly the calf muscles, is good for the feet; supple joints allow easy rocking across the bottom of the foot, and well-conditioned calf muscles help pull up the foot. One of the best ways to strengthen feet and keep them in shape is walking—not meandering, mind you, but brisk walks with long strides. When you walk, don't just slap your foot down. Roll through the whole foot, landing on your heel and using your toes to push off. Wear soft, thick socks and walking shoes that support and cushion your heel.

Here are a few specific foot-strengthening and foot-relaxation exercises.

♦ Walk barefoot. It stimulates the reflexes of the feet. To give your feet even more of a workout, walk on grass or sand or small pebbles. You can even tiptoe through the tulips.

♦ With your shoes off alternately point and flex your foot. Work each foot ten times.

♦ Stand up, still with your shoes off, and lift yourself up on tiptoe for a moment. (Keep your ankles and knees together so that your feet don't roll to the side.) Go back to normal stance for a moment and then back to your toes again. Repeat ten times.

♦ Put a squash ball or a small bottle under your foot and roll it back and forth for a few minutes. This relaxes feet that are tired from walking or other exercise.

FOOT MASSAGE

"When I see the foot, I see the whole body. Feet talk to me." That's what Rose Marie Martin, the Canyon Ranch reflexologist, is likely to answer if you ask her how she can tell if you have a stiff neck when she hasn't gone anywhere near it. One way or another she's had hundreds of conversations with feet.

As we explained in the last chapter, reflexology is based on the principle that the foot is divided into 10 zones, and each of the zones corresponds to another part of the body. By gently manipulating and massaging only the feet a reflexologist can give what basically amounts to a full body massage. Foot massage improves circulation (your whole body feels warm after just a few moments of having your feet massaged) and relieves tension, and it may be used to ease a string of ailments, including headaches, backaches, sinus problems, and asthma. It's no wonder that practically all massage therapists spend at least some time on the feet.

Massaging the feet relaxes the whole body, but naturally it's especially wonderful for the feet. It does a lot for speeding up the healing process of sprains and breaks. When fitness director Karma Kientzler broke her toe, she was told by her doctor that she wouldn't be able to walk on it for at least a week, but after two reflexology sessions in two days she was up and around.

HOW TO GIVE YOURSELF A FOOT-RUB

The study of reflexology takes a long time, and we're certainly not going to try to make a reflexologist out of you here. We do suggest, however, that you take a break now and then to give your feet a mini-massage. Be sure to keep it nice and simple; even five or ten minutes on each foot (finish with one before moving on to the other) will give you a new lease on life.

For best results you'll need some sort of cream or oil (Rose Marie Martin uses Nivea cream). Start with the big toe, working it firmly on the sides, top, and especially the ball and spending several minutes there before moving on to the ball of your foot. Next stop, the arch, and then comes the heel—both sides as well as the fleshier part. Now move to the instep and, finally, go back to the toes. Give each one at least 30 seconds of massage, going up and down the sides and then working the ball of each toe. If you like, finish with a soak in warm water and Epsom salts.

HOME REMEDIES

Doctoring your own feet can be a dangerous business, and generally we're dead set against it. Bunions, ingrown toenails, and plantar warts definitely require the attention of a podiatrist. But there are a few things you can do yourself without doing any harm:

♦ Soak tired, achy feet in Epsom salts and warm water. Sometimes the old ways are truly the best ways.

♦ If you do get a blister, prick it in several places with a sterilized needle, apply an antibiotic ointment, and cover it with a sterile dressing. If there is blood in the blister, see a doctor.

♦ Treating corns yourself can be a mistake. There is no harm in trying a corn plaster, but leave cutting and sanding to a professional.

♦ Athlete's foot. It's hard to cure athlete's foot forever, but one way to keep it under control is to wear cotton socks and shoes made of natural materials such as cotton and leather; they let feet breathe. Another is to dust your shoes with cornstarch before and after wearing to absorb moisture.

A FEW WORDS ABOUT HANDS

Most of us are lucky; our hands don't actually hurt. And because they don't hurt, we don't notice them very much. We certainly don't take time to find out how good they can really feel. The same reflexes that are in the foot are in the hands too, which means that manipulating the hands and exercising them can make the rest of us feel great. Massaging the hands is one of the nicest things you can do for yourself.

Get in the habit of working with your hands. Molding clay is terrific for the hands (one of the many things people enjoy about our Creative Arts Workshop), and so are working in the garden and playing with a vise grip you keep next to the telephone. When you're watching television or lying in the bath, do some hand exercises: stretch your hands out as far as they can go, then bend them back toward your body; then make circles with both hands, first one way and then the other. Touch each fingertip in turn to the tip of your thumb, making an O. Place your elbows and palms together and stretch out the fingers of each hand. Release the stretch and repeat several times.

And try this relaxing routine at least once a day. Using the thumb and forefinger of your right hand, gently massage each finger of the left. Start at the base of the finger and work your way toward the nails. Use your thumb to knead the palm of your hand and the upper part of your wrist. Switch hands, massaging your right hand with your left.

COMPLETING THE PICTURE

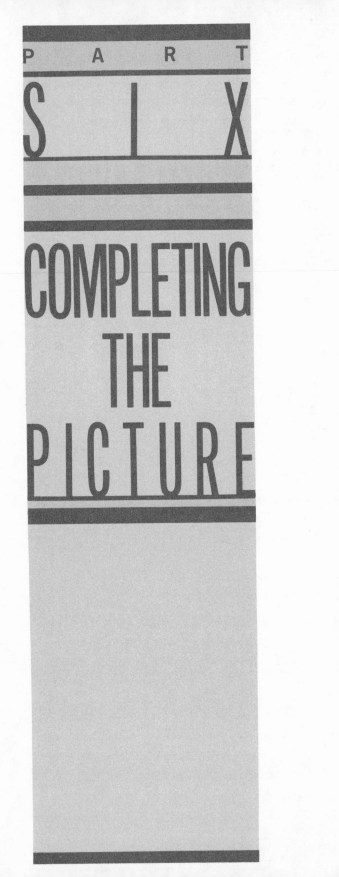

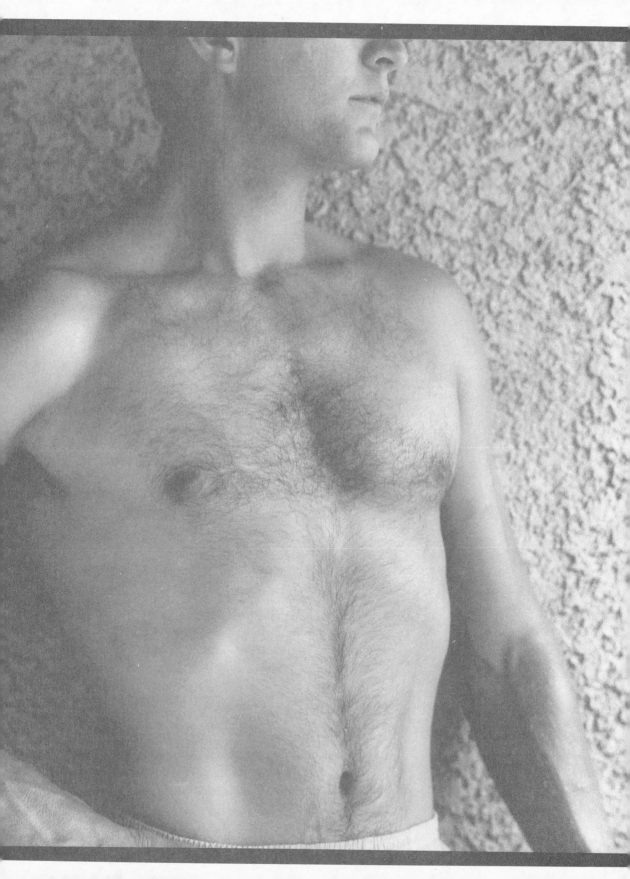

22

Sometimes—when you're at 35,000 feet and have been traveling for 11 hours, or when it's 10 o'clock at night and you've only just found the time to call room service for your dinner, or when you're in a wonderful new restaurant that specializes in Fat à la Mode and everyone around you is stuffing his face—fitness can be a real pain. Eating well and exercising regularly are not always easy when you're surrounded by the comforts of home, to be sure, but they're murder when you're not. Nutritionists at the University of Kansas Medical Center made it official; data they collected showed that frequent business travelers tend to eat a diet about 45 percent higher in fat than people who stay home.

In several earlier chapters (especially Chapters 6, 14, and 15) we touched on the subject of eating and exercising when you're out and about, but since it is such an important issue (it's the single biggest problem that our guests face), we'll focus a bit more on it here.

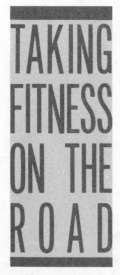

TAKING FITNESS ON THE ROAD

AIR TRAVEL

"When people get on planes, it's as if they move to another planet. Even if they normally are very sensible about what they eat, they immediately grab for a cocktail and a bag of peanuts and anything else the flight attendant hands them. And the problem is, all that stuff just makes people feel worse. Some people take days to feel normal again after taking a plane trip."

Fitness Director Karma Kientzler is talking about one of her favorite subjects: fitness on the road. In her thousands of counseling sessions with guests over the last nine years, it's the problem she has heard about most, so she has made it her business to become something of an expert.

When she gives advice, the thrust of the message she gives is this: if you think ahead and do a little planning, you do not have to be at the mercy of airlines, hotels, waiters, or business colleagues. Armed with motivation and the following Rules of the Road, you can stay in charge of your life.

RULE #1. KNOW YOUR BODY'S RHYTHMS

You know whether you're a morning or an evening person, but you may not be taking that knowledge seriously enough when you travel. Don't fight your body's rhythms; work around them. If you are more comfortable traveling in the morning, do so. If you like to travel at night but your meeting is very early in the morning, think about going the day before. A hotel room for an extra night may seem extravagant, but if your trip is very long, you may well need the time to rest and get your bearings. To make adjustments to a new time zone a little easier, adjust your watch as soon as you get on the plane. The sooner you stop thinking about what time it "really" is, the better.

RULE #2. EAT AND DRINK SENSIBLY

It's a lot easier to eat sensibly on planes than it used to be. Many airlines have relatively healthful alternatives to Mystery Meat: fruit platters, vegetarian and kosher meals, fish dinners, and low-cal, low-sodium, and low-fat platters. If you must eat on planes—Karma recommends against it, suggesting that you're much better off fueling your body before you travel and after you get there—your best bets are the fish or fruit. To avoid having to eat what is put in front of you, carry a banana, an orange, or an apple with you.

You don't really need food on a plane, but because travel is extremely dehydrating (the constipation and fatigue that often accompany travel result mostly from dehydration), you do need liquid, preferably water or seltzer. Coffee, tea, soft drinks, and any sort of alcohol make you even more dehydrated.

RULE #3. PICK THE RIGHT HOTEL

One of our guests, a woman who travels on business for about two weeks out of every month lost 20 pounds in three months by having lunch in her hotel room instead of in a restaurant. Of course, she picked the right hotel, one that had a good room service menu and let her rent an exercise bike and a videocassette player for her room. Instead of having a glass of wine and a full meal at midday she cycled and worked out to a stretch tape for 45 minutes and then ate a fruit plate.

There are many such accommodating hotels these days, since the demand for health-conscious lodgings has increased greatly over the last ten years. Many have pools and other sports facilities, or, if they don't, they may be able to help you work out a deal with a nearby health club. If you're a regular guest of a hotel that doesn't offer much in the way of fitness equipment, try to persuade the manager to invest in a treadmill, rowing machine, or exercise bike that you can rent during your stay. If you don't have any luck with that request, think about buying one yourself and asking the hotel to keep it in storage for you.

RULE #4. TAKE ADVANTAGE OF LAYOVERS

One of the best places to have a layover (technically a wait of three hours or more) is Dallas, because the airport there has an honest-to-goodness fitness facility. Instead of killing time eating barbecued beef, you can get a full workout. If you have a layover, give the airport where you'll be cooling your heels a call and ask what, if any, facilities it has. If it doesn't have any (unfortunately, most don't), ask if there is a nearby hotel where you can take a swim or ride an exercise bike for a while or take a shower after you jog. Many airport hotels, aware that there is a market here, allow you to work out in their facilities for a fee; some even provide gym clothes and other equipment. If all else fails, travel in your jogging shoes. Between planes check your bags and walk the airport.

RULE #5. PACK FOR FITNESS

Tennis shoes, squash shoes, running shoes, goggles, bathing suit, bathing cap, jogging gear, dumbbells, jump rope, shorts, leotards, tights, sweats, cycling helmet, exercise mat—it would be great to take all of that and more with you wherever you go. Obviously you can't, especially if you need to travel light. Even if space is at a premium, however, you should take the clothes you need for two kinds of activities. In case of rain, you probably won't be able to run, but you can swim in the pool or take an aerobics class. (Karma, who spent most of the first 16 years of her life in a swimming pool, says that even if swimming is not your fitness activity of choice, you should travel with a swimsuit. Paddling around in the water is a great comfort, something many of us especially need when we're away from home.)

Most people can get along with athletic shoes, a couple of pairs of good socks (one light and one athletic), a pair of shorts, a T-shirt, sweats, and—most important—a waterproof bag for packing damp workout clothes.

RULE #6. LEARN HOW TO RELAX

Karma says she's no fun at all as a traveling companion, since she sleeps all the time she's on the plane. A few years ago she learned how to use self-hypnosis to will herself to sleep almost the minute the plane left the ground. You don't have to sleep your travel time away, of course, but you'll have a healthier and happier time of it if you find something to do—besides eat and drink, that is—that will keep you from getting bored, tense, or anxious. In Chapter 17 we described stress management techniques, many of which will serve you well in the air. Breathing, meditation, and progressive relaxation are particularly good. So are reading a book, playing cards, and doing anything else that occupies your hands and mind.

RULE #7. RIDE IN COMFORT

When Karma isn't snoozing on a plane, she's moving around, stretching in her seat, strolling in the aisles, and generally trying to make up for the fact that airline seats are designed for safe takeoffs and landings, not for ergonomics. Traveling is rough on all the joints, but it's particularly hard on the back. Most airlines provide small pillows, so grab a couple of them before takeoff, one for behind your neck and the other for your lower back. Don't make your spine conform to the seat; maintain the natural curve of your spine. If there's a chance there won't be any pillows on the flight, think about investing in a couple of small inflatable pillows.

When you're in the air, keep your back and the rest of your body loose by doing some easy, fairly unobtrusive stretching exercises. Every half-hour or so sit up straight and turn around and look over your shoulder, lengthening your body through the torso. This improves your circulation as well as keeping you supple. Don't cross your legs if you can avoid it, but if you must, at least alternate the crossed legs regularly. Each time you switch sides do a few ankle circles, first clockwise, then counterclockwise. To expand your lungs and loosen your neck and shoulder muscles, lift your arms over your head and hold your right elbow with your left hand and your left elbow with your right. Lift yourself up and take a deep breath. On long flights every hour or so take a stroll around the plane and stretch. For maximum comfort wear loose clothing made of natural fabrics and comfortable (preferably athletic) shoes.

RULE #8. TAKE TIME TO EXERCISE

If you're in good shape, exercising every other day should be plenty, but if you have weight to lose, you'll need to get some sort of aerobic workout at least five times a week. No matter what shape you're in, if you don't exercise when you travel, you're asking for trouble, since inactivity usually leads to overeating and excessive drinking, which usually leads to more inactivity. You simply can't afford to take a vacation from fitness. You have to find a way to move your body.

If you need some inspiration, think about the couple who spent three weeks in Africa last year. For about 18 months before their safari they had been jogging four times a week, and they really wanted to keep it up. For obvious reasons they were nervous about running alone in the bush, so they hired a jeep and driver to follow them along their route every morning. Jeeps and drivers may seem a bit much, but the moral of the story applies to everyone; if you have the will to stay fit on the road, you can find a way.

RULE #9. BE GOOD TO YOURSELF

As we've said many times, there is more to fitness than eating right and getting regular exercise. You also have to take time out to pamper yourself a little. One excellent way to ease the stress of traveling is to treat yourself to an herbal bath when you get to your room. (Steep four or five tea bags in a hot bath and relax in it for 20 minutes.) Mint is particularly nice for post-travel relaxation, since it stimulates the surface of the skin and clears the sinuses. If you have trouble sleeping, drink some herbal tea; chamomile is a particularly pleasant soporific. Get into the habit of including tea bags in your travel kit. For a special treat, see if you can get a massage in the hotel before bed.

How to Survive in Restaurants

You know the drill by heart. For your appetizer you'll have clear broth; no creamed soups or clams casino will pass your lips. Then you'll probably have broiled fish, but if you choose chicken or meat, you'll have it roasted, baked, broiled, grilled, or poached, not fried or breaded. Potatoes will be baked, boiled, or steamed, hold the butter and sour cream. You'll have lemon juice or mustard. To go along with that you'll have steamed vegetables and a plain salad, please. All sauces, gravies, and dressings will be served, if at all, on the side. When the dessert cart comes around, you'll have the fruit.

But then you get to the restaurant, and your plans go up in smoke. You're ravenous when you get there, and there's a huge bread basket on the table. A couple of the people in your party are late, so you have a drink and a piece of bread. Then you have another drink and another piece of bread and somebody suggests ordering a few appetizers while you wait for the others, maybe some fried zucchini or stuffed mushrooms. The appetizers get there, your glass is empty, you still haven't ordered your meal, and you're starting to get the distinct impression that life isn't fair. If your friends can eat all this food, why oh why can't you? So you do.

And to think that restaurant dining is supposed to be fun!

Actually it can be fun, but only if you don't end up feeling deprived or guilty or, as is usually the case, both. In order not to let that happen you have to have a Plan.

STRATEGIES FOR DINING OUT

In Chapters 14 and 15 we talked at length about ways of changing your diet and managing your eating habits, all of which serve you well whether you're eating in your kitchen or in a four-star restaurant. However, here are a few strategies that are particularly useful when you're dining out.

♦ Don't arrive ravenous. An apple or a couple of crackers can come between you and a bowl of peanuts.

♦ Educate yourself about how foods are prepared and what kinds of satisfactions different foods give you. Fish filets and tomato slices are wonderful, but they're not chewy, so if chewy is what you need, they won't be enough. When you're not sure how a dish is prepared, ask your waiter. If the menu doesn't include any obvious choices for you, ask the waiter to find out what the chef recommends as a low-fat entrée.

♦ If you know exactly what you want but don't think you have the strength to say the words, write down your order and hand it to the waiter or to your dinner companion. If you're feeling very weak and susceptible to temptation, excuse yourself from the table when others are ordering.

♦ Eat the best and skip the rest. If what you really want is soup, salad, and one of those great-looking desserts, you should probably have exactly that. Having broiled fish and a plain salad will just make you unhappy and frustrated, and you'll probably end up having one of those great-looking desserts anyhow. Be creative in your meal planning. There's no law that says you have to order an appetizer, a main course, and a dessert.

♦ Watch out for portion sizes. Servings in most restaurants are much too large, particularly when it comes to meat and other protein sources. If you are served more than you want to eat, there are several things you can do to keep from eating the whole thing: you can use your willpower and ignore it; you can ask your waiter to take away your plate and bring back half; or you can render half of the meal inedible by oversalting it. Do whatever you think is necessary. Paying full price for a half-portion may seem expensive, but you'll pay dearly in other ways if you eat more than you want to eat.

♦ Keep your hands busy. Idle hands often end up rooting around in the bread basket. Be aware of the "play" value of many foods; they take time and energy to eat. Some of the best are artichokes, corn on the cob, paella, cioppino, bouillabaisse, lobster, mussels, and clams.

♦ Don't let starches scare you. There are worse things to eat than a breadstick or a piece of bread, as long as it's not loaded with butter. Better unbuttered bread than nuts, fried zucchini, or potato chips.

◆ If you decide to have a drink, have it with your meal or even afterward. A glass of wine can make a very nice dessert.

WHAT TO ORDER

Many people feel that there are some kinds of restaurants that are off-limits to them when they're watching their weight. While there may be some truth to that—if you know that you can't control yourself when it comes to Indian food, for instance, you probably are better off going somewhere else—you can find something nutritious to order in virtually all restaurants if you know what you're doing. Here are a few tips.

◆ Seafood. Avoid New England clam chowder, fried fish, anything stuffed, clams casino, and lobster Newburg. Choose shellfish in the shell, grilled shrimp and scallops, or poached or grilled fillets.

◆ Steakhouses. The reason that filet mignon, delmonico steak, and New York steaks are so tender and juicy is that they contain a lot of fat. Choose London broil and eat half of whatever you're served. The normal portion of steak is eight to ten ounces.

◆ Mexican. As you can imagine, we love this kind of food in Tucson. But we make the right choices: soft tortillas with salsa, seviche, tamales, bean burritos, black beans, rice, tostados, and bean entrées. The problems are large portions and fried foods: nachos, guacamole, sour cream, refried beans, and fried tortillas (soft tortillas are baked).

◆ Italian. There are lots of good choices here: minestrone, anything *marinara,* red clam sauce, chicken cacciatore, veal piccata, and lots of pasta. Watch out for cheese sauces, breading, and cream, which means no lasagna, fettucine Alfredo, or anything *parmigiana.* Since portions are often large, think about ordering side dishes as entrées.

◆ Chinese. Watch out for the word *fried* unless it's preceded by the word *stir-*: fried rice, fried noodles, deep-fried egg rolls, fried dumplings. Avoid pork and sweet-and-sour entrées or anything with nuts. Have soups, bean curd entrées, or stir-fried chicken or shrimp with lots of vegetables and rice. If you eat family style, serve yourself in the bowl that the rice comes in and eat one course at a time.

◆ Cajun. Order steamed crawfish, shrimp steamed in beer, broiled redfish or salmon, collards, and red beans. Avoid cajun popcorn and shrimp fritters, gumbo, blackened redfish, cornsticks, and hushpuppies.

◆ French. Say *non* to duck, pastry shells, heavy cream, and calorie-laden sauces, such as béarnaise, béchamel, and mornay. Choose coulis or piquante instead. Best bets: bouillabaisse, chicken, and fish or seafood entrées with sauce on the side.

♦ Diners. The great American foods—chicken-fried steak, croquettes, biscuits and gravy, macaroni and cheese, tuna casseroles—are loaded with fat and calories. Your best bet is white meat turkey (gravy on the side) and salad.

♦ Delis. The delicatessen's stock in trade, processed meats and cheeses with a side order of potato salad or cole slaw, is a deadly mix—almost all fat. The best sandwich is sliced chicken or turkey on whole wheat with lettuce, tomato, and mustard. Even better, have half a sandwich.

♦ Pizza. Stay away from meat toppings and double cheese and pile on the vegetables instead. Since the crust is better for you than the cheese, have one piece of thick-crust pizza instead of two slices of thin.

♦ Salad bars. Avoid egg, cheese, meats, bacon bits, nuts and seeds, blue cheese dressings, potato and macaroni salad. Choose the vegetables that are not sitting in oil.

♦ Fast food. This may as well be called *fat* food. If you must indulge, choose plain burgers, stuffed spuds (without cheese), pita pocket sandwiches, or salads.

SPLURGING

One of the strategies that Julie Kembel recommends is one or two "free" restaurant meals a month, occasions when you give yourself permission to eat whatever you want. She has found that since people overeat once in a while anyway, they may as well make it part of their grand design. If you don't let up on yourself every once in a while, she says, you may rebel by giving up on the plan altogether.

SURVIVING SPECIAL OCCASIONS

'Tis the season to be jolly. 'Tis also the season to put on five or ten pounds, skip exercising, drink too much, and eat foods you haven't even thought about in a year. Sometimes it seems that what really makes these occasions special is that you lose control, make yourself miserable, and hate yourself in the morning.

Unfortunately fitness is not always festive, but that does not mean that you can't enjoy cocktail parties and birthday celebrations and Thanksgiving dinner as much as the next guy. You just need a realistic attitude and, again, a Plan.

The attitude is fairly simple to explain; first, don't try to lose weight when all around you are doing their best to gain it; be satisfied just to maintain your weight, whatever it is. Second, begin to think of holiday celebrations and other festivities as pleasant occasions that are not about food. Focus on the people who will be there and the activities other than eating that you can enjoy. Plan to dance all night or get a game of charades or touch football going. Get a group together to look at the family scrapbook or walk the dog. Take everybody bowling. There are plenty of things you can do to enjoy the company of your friends and family besides eating fudge. Third, understand that times of celebrations are also times of stress, and brace yourself for it. Be ready too for a little social pressure; someone probably slaved all day on that fudge, and she may be hurt if you don't try it. If you give in, you are letting someone else take charge of your life.

As always, the best way to prevent loss of control is to plan ahead; if you know what to expect, you can avoid the pitfalls. Here are a few things that usually work:

♦ Don't skip meals, but do "bank" your calories a little. Eating just a little less at a few meals before the big occasion gives you some much-needed leeway.

♦ Don't arrive at a party hungry.

♦ If it's all right with your host, take something to the party that you can comfortably eat. If you don't eat anything, you'll feel deprived and may react by overeating later. Ask if you can contribute a vegetable tray; most hosts would be glad to serve one without having to do all the peeling and chopping themselves.

♦ Keep exercising. This can be difficult during the holidays—we're all too busy having fun to stay fit—but it's crucial. A late afternoon workout can be very helpful in getting you through an evening of parties without overindulging, but the problem is, if you wait until late, the day may get away from you and you may not do it at all. The best strategy seems to be to do your exercise first thing in the morning and get it *done*.

THE MORNING AFTER

Whatever you do, don't weigh yourself the day after you've overeaten or drunk too much and don't spend the day flogging yourself over your excesses. As we discussed in Chapter 15, when you overindulge, go back to "first position." Have your regular breakfast, get your regular amount of exercise, and regain your balance. Don't pretend that last night never happened; if you do, you won't have learned anything to help you next time. And as long as there are parties, there *will* be a next time.

23

There are ten people in the small, sunny room, and more than a few of them look completely miserable. Although the room is air-conditioned, one man has broken out into a sweat. A few people seem to have the sniffles. Almost everyone is fidgeting. One woman who can't sit still paces at the back of the room. Someone cracks a joke, but only half the people in the room laugh, and a little nervously at that. The others seem to have lost their sense of humor. It looks like something out of *The Manchurian Candidate*, but it's not. It's Day 1 of the Canyon Ranch Stop Smoking Program.

That description is an exaggeration—at least a little—and the misery that it depicts is only temporary. In fact, by the end of the four-day program the scene will have changed dramatically. Granted, the group still won't be as relaxed and cheerful as the people playing Wallyball, learning how to make quesadillas, or watching the evening movie, but they'll be feeling better, much better.

Along the way they will have learned that the discomfort they've been feeling is all for a very good cause. Nothing you can do for your health, not even dieting or exercise or stress management or a month-long vacation, pays off more quickly than giving up smoking. In Chapter 3 we gave you the bad news—a checklist of all the terrible things that smoking does to your heart, lungs, and other body parts. Here's the good news. A few nicotine-free years can put you back in the non-smokers' category as far as most health risks are concerned. Within two years of your quitting, smoking will cease to be a risk factor for heart disease. Within ten years your risk of lung cancer will be the same as that of someone who never smoked at all. Within 20 minutes your blood

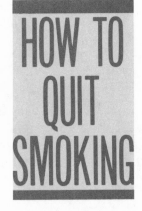

HOW TO QUIT SMOKING

pressure will drop, your heart rate will decrease, and your circulation will be better. Before too long you'll sleep a lot better, and your skin will look healthier. Sure, you'll feel cranky for a while, but it will be worth it.

Being Ready to Quit

In the time we spend with our Stop Smoking guests we try to teach a lot of things, but we also learn, encouraging our pupils to talk about why they smoke and why they feel ready to quit. In a class we might hear any one or more of the following: "My best friend just died of lung cancer"; I'm tired of feeling like a leper"; "My doctor says if I don't bring my blood pressure down, I'll have a heart attack in six months"; "I've been having chest pains"; "I'm sick of being a slave to a habit—I want to get back in control"; "My husband says he'll leave me if I don't quit"; "My company has just started a no-smoking policy"; and "It's a disgusting habit." At any session the reasons we hear are as dramatic as the fear of death or as seemingly mundane as not wanting to get the worst table in a restaurant.

Everyone who smokes has some or all of those feelings some or all of the time, but having the feelings doesn't necessarily mean that you're psychologically ready to quit. (In fact, some of the people in the program are there to "audit" the course, as part of the getting-ready process.) Quite simply put, you are ready to quit smoking when your reasons for breaking the habit outweigh your desire to smoke. Wanting to do it is the key to success. The next step is a willingness to invest as much time and energy in your nonsmoking behavior as you did in your smoking behavior.

Saying Goodbye to a Friend

The phone rings, and you reach for your cigarettes. You turn the key in the ignition of your car, and it's time to light up. Holding a cocktail or a cup of coffee in one hand without a cigarette in the other is unthinkable. Let's face it—you and your cigarettes have developed a meaningful relationship. It's no exaggeration to say that some smokers are more attached to their cigarettes than they are to almost anything else in their lives. It's easy to understand why. Day after day, smoking is always there, always dependable. In times of happiness or pain or joy or frustration, you can always light up a cigarette.

Giving that up is by no means easy. Many people who give up cigarettes experience a real sense of loss, almost grief. Some go through a genuine period of mourning. One four-pack-a-day smoker was so upset when he quit that he commemorated the death of his habit with a funeral. He buried his cigarettes, matches, lighters, and even his favorite coffee cup in a box in the garden.

WHY WE SMOKE

Why do you smoke? This is a hard question for many smokers to answer, and many don't particularly enjoy the soul-searching process. "What difference does it make why I do it?" they say. "All I care about is quitting!" Alas, it's not that simple. Human nature is such that it is easier to break a habit if we can replace it with something else. For every reason we smoke there is probably a behavior we can substitute that will go a long way toward easing the pain. A cigarette is a tool that helps us cope. It is better to have a different tool than to do without.

It's possible you won't even remember what prompted you to light up a cigarette for the first time. Maybe you were in high school, and you wanted to feel cool. Perhaps you were in the service, and everybody else was doing it. One woman started smoking after her first baby was born. The infant was colicky, and every time the baby cried, she'd light up a cigarette. After a few months the baby's colic went away, but by then she was up to three packs a day.

Habitual smokers do it because they like the taste, because it relaxes them, relieves pressure, lets them unwind, and gives them something to do with their hands. The smoking ritual—taking out the pack, removing the cigarette, putting it in the mouth, lighting up—buys them a minute or two of free time. People also smoke to rebel, to live dangerously, to break rules.

To get a better idea of what kind of tool a cigarette is for you, answer the questions on the following form (see page 242).

Now compute your score and see what it all means. Following the chart is a rough interpretation of the results and some suggestions about what you can do to replace the smoking habit with something a little less destructive. Bear in mind that this is not a science. No matter which kind of smoker you are, all of the "Recommended Substitute Behaviors" can be helpful to you in your efforts to quit.

WHY DO YOU SMOKE?

Here are some statements made by people to describe what they get out of smoking. How often do you feel this way about smoking? Circle one number for each statement.

		AL-WAYS	FRE-QUENTLY	OCCA-SION-ALLY	SEL-DOM	NEVER
A.	I SMOKE CIGARETTES IN ORDER TO KEEP MYSELF FROM SLOWING DOWN.	5	4	3	2	1
B.	HANDLING A CIGARETTE IS PART OF THE ENJOYMENT OF SMOKING IT.	5	4	3	2	1
C.	SMOKING CIGARETTES IS PLEASANT AND RELAXING.	5	4	3	2	1
D.	I LIGHT UP A CIGARETTE WHEN I FEEL ANGRY ABOUT SOMETHING.	5	4	3	2	1
E.	WHEN I HAVE RUN OUT OF CIGARETTES, I FIND IT ALMOST UNBEARABLE UNTIL I CAN GET THEM.	5	4	3	2	1
F.	I SMOKE CIGARETTES AUTOMATICALLY, WITHOUT EVEN BEING AWARE OF IT.	5	4	3	2	1
G.	I SMOKE CIGARETTES TO STIMULATE MY-SELF, TO PERK UP.	5	4	3	2	1
H.	PART OF THE ENJOYMENT OF SMOKING A CIGARETTE COMES FROM THE STEPS I TAKE TO LIGHT UP.	5	4	3	2	1
I.	I FIND CIGARETTES PLEASURABLE.	5	4	3	2	1
J.	WHEN I FEEL UNCOMFORTABLE OR UPSET ABOUT SOMETHING, I LIGHT UP A CIGA-RETTE.	5	4	3	2	1
K.	I AM VERY MUCH AWARE OF THE FACT WHEN I AM NOT SMOKING A CIGARETTE.	5	4	3	2	1
L.	I LIGHT UP A CIGARETTE WITHOUT REALIZ-ING I STILL HAVE ONE BURNING IN THE ASHTRAY.	5	4	3	2	1
M.	I SMOKE CIGARETTES TO GIVE ME A "LIFT."	5	4	3	2	1

	AL-WAYS	FRE-QUENTLY	OCCA-SION-ALLY	SEL-DOM	NEVER
N. WHEN I SMOKE A CIGARETTE, PART OF THE ENJOYMENT IS WATCHING THE SMOKE AS I EXHALE IT.	5	4	3	2	1
O. I WANT A CIGARETTE MOST WHEN I AM COMFORTABLE AND RELAXED.	5	4	3	2	1
P. WHEN I FEEL "BLUE" OR WANT TO TAKE MY MIND OFF CARES AND WORRIES, I SMOKE CIGARETTES.	5	4	3	2	1
Q. I GET A REAL GNAWING HUNGER FOR A CIGARETTE WHEN I HAVEN'T SMOKED FOR A WHILE.	5	4	3	2	1
R. I'VE FOUND A CIGARETTE IN MY MOUTH AND DIDN'T REMEMBER PUTTING IT THERE.	5	4	3	2	1

HOW TO SCORE:

1. Enter the number you have circled for each question in the spaces below, putting the number you have circled for Question A over line A, to Question B over Line B, etc.

					TOTALS
___ A	+	___ G	+	___ M	= ___ Stimulation
___ B	+	___ H	+	___ N	= ___ Handling
___ C	+	___ I	+	___ O	= ___ Pleasurable Relaxation
___ D	+	___ J	+	___ P	= ___ Crutch: Tension Reduction
___ E	+	___ K	+	___ Q	= ___ Craving: Psychological Addiction
___ F	+	___ L	+	___ R	= ___ Habit

◆ Stimulation. A high score here means that cigarettes energize you. They make you feel more alert, more animated, and better able to organize your thoughts. *Recommended Substitute Behavior:* Stay active. If you need stimulation, get up and move around, do some exercise, run an errand. If you feel like eating, make it something very crunchy or very spicy. Better yet, brush your teeth with a strongly flavored toothpaste or gargle with a strong mouthwash.

◆ Handling. Moderate to high scores in handling mean that you need something to keep your hands busy, especially when you're anxious or restless. *Recommended Substitute Behavior:* Never be without something to keep your hands occupied—worry beads, swizzle sticks, a jigsaw puzzle, something to doodle on. Take up needlepoint, polish the silver, do your nails, or wrap Christmas presents.

◆ Relaxation. Lots of people score high in this category, but it's hard to understand how anything that speeds up the heart rate and the metabolism could be considered relaxing. Of course, nicotine is not relaxing, but a cigarette is the vehicle around which many smokers relax themselves, thinking, "I'll relax and have a cigarette." The cigarette doesn't do it; *you* do. The cigarette is just a tool by which you give yourself permission to relax. *Recommended Substitute Behavior:* Unfortunately many people in this category substitute eating for smoking, not a particularly constructive substitution. Instead try deep breathing or massage to relax you. Take a bath, go to a movie, or go out dancing.

◆ Crutch. Some people are convinced that they absolutely can't get through a crisis or even a mildly difficult situation without a cigarette. "I can't believe this is happening. I'm a wreck. I need a cigarette to calm me down!" they say. Again it's not the cigarette that reduces tension or gets you through a rocky time. It's telling yourself that you will be calmed by it. *Recommended Substitute Behavior:* Slow, measured deep breathing can be a wonderful tranquilizer. So can yoga, the company of friends, and watching a favorite old movie.

◆ Craving. High scorers in this category often want the next cigarette even before the last one has been stubbed out. *Recommended Substitute Behavior:* In some ways this is the most difficult of all. Although the average cigarette craving lasts only 30 to 90 seconds, it can seem like forever. Plan distractions that will keep you occupied while it goes away. Take each craving one at a time.

◆ Habit. These are the smokers who are forever leaving their cigarettes burning in the ashtray, forgetting that they're even there. They need to light their cigarettes more than they need to smoke them. *Recommended Substitute Behavior:* Change your patterns, so that you no longer associate smoking with other activities. If you are used to smoking when you talk on the phone, move the phone to another spot and leave a Rubik's Cube or a lump of modeling clay next to it. Spend more time around nonsmokers.

WITHDRAWAL—BODY AND MIND

Let's go back to all those cranky, fidgety people we described at the beginning of the chapter. Are they just chronic malcontents, or do they have a good reason to feel rotten? They have a *great* reason. Smoking is an extremely strong chemical addiction (the Surgeon General made it official in May of 1988); some say that a nicotine habit is harder to kick than even heroin or cocaine. When you stop smoking, your body must readjust to a normal state in which it no longer needs nicotine. This is a process that your body does not enjoy, to say the least, and it pays you back—in the short term, anyway—with any one or more of the following maladies: headaches, nausea, dizziness, mood swings, agitation, fatigue, drowsiness, muscle cramps, and constipation. Nicotine withdrawal can also disturb your sleep, make you cough, and leave you disoriented, scatterbrained, and depressed. To make matters even worse, it makes you hungry. It's no wonder the people in the Stop Smoking class aren't having much fun.

Of course, not everyone in the class is suffering equally; some lucky souls have it much easier than others, and for some the real physical suffering is over quite quickly. Physical withdrawal symptoms last for about a week, or two weeks at the most. The worst is over after about four days. The urge to smoke will last longer, but it too will become less intense as time goes on. (We've heard stories of people who don't crave cigarettes during the waking hours but find themselves lighting up in their dreams.)

How many people do you know who have quit smoking for six months, a year, even five years, and gone back to the habit? This has nothing to do with a physical craving for a cigarette; it has to do with the emotional crutch that a cigarette represents. If the physical addiction to cigarettes is a formidable thing, the psychological addiction is awesome. (In the four-day program we spend one on the former and the rest of the time on the latter.) Always remember that in addition to being a nicotine source a cigarette is a tool. Like a shovel or a cheese grater or a word processor, it helps you to accomplish a job. Even when you no longer want a cigarette, you want what the cigarette does for you.

THE 13-STEP PROGRAM

Here's the short version of what we talk about in Stop Smoking. If you're seriously considering cutting out cigarettes, follow the program closely. We guarantee that it will go easier on you.

1   Do your homework. Think about what kind of smoker you are. Keep a smoking diary for a week or so, recording how much and when you smoke, what else you were doing at the time, and how you felt. Look for patterns in your smoking behavior. Understand that you use a cigarette as a coping tool and think about other tools that might take its place. Be specific.

2   Make a list. Write down the reasons you want to quit smoking. Keep it nearby and review it often.

3   Set the date. Pick a day that you're going to quit and stick to your schedule. The best choice is probably a weekend (not a holiday) when you'll be under relatively little stress and you have a flexible schedule. If you're having a crisis in your life, settle it first. Remember, though, if you wait until there is absolutely nothing else going on in your life before you quit, it will never happen.

4   Take it one day at a time. One of the things that scares people most is thinking, "I can never have another cigarette as long as I live." It's hard to imagine that the time will come when you won't even think about smoking, but it will. In the meantime, don't think about next year; focus all your attention on not smoking today.

5   Spread the word. Tell the world that you've quit smoking. Make your friends, family, and co-workers congratulate you, feel sorry for you, and give you support. There are nearly as many former smokers in this country today as there are current smokers, and every one of them absolutely loves to talk about kicking the habit. Talk to them.

6   Get help. It's comforting to know that there are plenty of people in the world who want you to quit smoking almost as much as you do. Hospitals, community organizations, the American Cancer Society, and the American Lung Association have free or low-cost programs. There are plenty of commercial programs too, which use hypnosis, aversion therapy (sometimes using electric shock, which can elevate your blood pressure), or behavior modification. If you need some help, investigate the available programs and pick one that seems best to you. If you want to stop badly enough, any system will work, including no system at all.

7   Clean house. A formal burial for your smoking paraphernalia may seem a bit much, but you should definitely get rid of anything

associated with the habit. Throw out cigarettes, lighters, and ash-trays. Have your teeth cleaned and your clothes laundered. Get a facial and shampoo the rugs. Remove all traces of your smoking habit from your home, office, and car.

8 Work up a sweat. The more you sweat, the faster the nicotine will leave your body. Naturally, vigorous exercise works well here, but so do saunas, steam, whirlpool baths, herbal baths and wraps, and inhalation therapy. Drinking plenty of water helps too.

9 Look for "no smoking" areas. Spend time in museums, movie theaters, department stores, health clubs, libraries, churches, and any other place you're used to being without a cigarette. Stay away from smokers.

10 Exercise. Aerobic exercise will help you keep from gaining weight and remind you of how much better you feel now that you've quit. Another benefit of exercise is that you can't possibly smoke while you do it. Swim, jog, ride a bike, play tennis, anything you like.

11 Reward yourself. Do something that will make you feel better: take a golf lesson, make an appointment for a massage (jin shin is especially good), sleep on flannel sheets, go to a ballgame, take in a movie with your friends.

12 Learn how to relax. Your days of relaxing with a cigarette are over, so you have to learn stress reduction techniques that will take the place of smoking. We highly recommend deep breathing, relaxation yoga, meditation, and hypnotherapy, but you don't have to opt for an "official" relaxation technique. It can be anything from climbing a mountain to curling up with a good mystery.

13 Count your blessings. Take time out from feeling sorry for yourself to compute how much money you're saving and enjoy the fact that no one is giving you dirty looks in restaurants anymore. Revel in the knowledge that you'll never again have to go out in the rain in the middle of the night because you've run out of smokes. Picture your lungs and heart.

THE NO-SMOKING DIET

You'll notice that in the preceding list of tips we didn't list one that says, "Eat everything you can get your hands on." Unfortunately, however, that's precisely what you're inclined to do when you give up smoking, partly because food tends to taste better than usual but mostly out of a desire to put something between your lips besides a cigarette. What's more, your metabolic rate goes down when you quit smoking; it is estimated that smoking burns as many as 250 calories a day. Between the overeating and the under-burning it's normal to gain between five and ten pounds when you quit.

There's no use going around complaining that life isn't fair and no good deed goes unpunished, although it's certainly tempting to do so. It's also a temptation to use weight gain as an excuse to start smoking again. It would be wonderful to say that there's a magic formula for avoiding weight gain when you quit smoking, but there isn't. The only solution to the problem is to eat a little more carefully and exercise a little more vigorously. For advice on how to do both turn to Part II (Moving Your Body) and Part III (Feeding Your Body).

There are a few tips that can keep you from piling on the pounds when you cut out cigarettes:

♦ Drink lots of water, mineral water, and juice. They help flush toxins from your system more quickly.

♦ When you nibble (and you will), choose high-chew or very crunchy low-cal foods.

♦ Stock up on cinnamon sticks. They give you something to play with and suck on, and they even have a hole in the middle so you can "inhale" the cinnamon taste. Minted toothpicks are handy too.

♦ Learn how to choose the right foods and manage your food habits. (See Chapters 14 and 15.)

THE "MODIFIED COLD TURKEY" METHOD

The prospect of cutting out cigarettes is so daunting that some smokers choose instead to cut down, smoking progressively less over time until they eventually quit altogether. We don't recommend the "modified cold turkey" method, only because the success rate doesn't appear to be as high as it does when you quit the old-fashioned way. If for some reason you decide to go this route, however, be sure you're methodical about it. Simply saying that you're going to cut down won't work. You have to have a plan—to be completely off cigarettes in 30 days, for instance. The following should help you formulate one and carry it out.

♦ Buy one pack at a time.

♦ Smoke a brand you don't like.

♦ Forget switching to low-tar cigarettes, cigars, or pipes. They can be just as risky as cigarettes (with low-tar cigarettes you drag harder and longer), and they don't appear to improve the success rate.

♦ Store cigarettes in a hard-to-get-at place—a plastic bag in the freezer, for instance.

♦ Postpone lighting your first cigarette of the day by five minutes the first day and an additional five minutes every day after that.

◆ Set aside nonsmoking hours every day.

◆ Change your routine. Go places where you don't usually smoke. Don't sit in your "smoking" chair.

◆ Give up coffee and cocktails for a while.

◆ After a meal smoke half a cigarette and quickly leave the table and brush your teeth.

◆ Chart your progress. Don't destroy the evidence by emptying ashtrays.

COPING WITH SETBACKS

Every year three million people quit smoking, and most of them are not doing it for the first time. National figures say that it takes three tries before you quit for good. What makes us try and fail? Almost anything. When it comes to inventing excuses to have a cigarette ("just one" we tell ourselves, lying through our teeth), we're veritable geniuses. When you're under a lot of stress, an "I don't care" attitude can crop up. Crises seem to cry out for a cigarette. You light one up, forgetting for the moment that smoking actually increases stress. (So does the knowledge that now you have to quit all over again.) Then there's "I deserve it" and "Why should I give up everything I like?" and "This is a special occasion." Try to remember that a cigarette is many things, but it is not a celebration. Find new ways to commemorate your joy.

No matter how strong your resolve is, there are times when you're particularly vulnerable to slip-ups. When you're drinking, when you're tired and crabby, when you feel off balance and out of control, when you're playing poker with the guys or ringing in the New Year at the club—all of these situations and more can offer what seem like perfect excuses to have "just one" cigarette.

Do everything you can to keep from having that first cigarette, but if you do give in, don't regard a mistake as failure; smoking one cigarette doesn't mean you're a smoker again. Don't let it ruin you. Learn from your mistakes, set a new date, grab your worry beads and your cinnamon sticks, and start again.

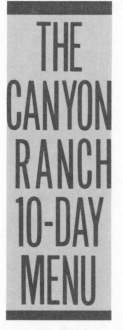

24

Everybody loves Day 10 at Canyon Ranch. That's when we serve the Canyon Ranch Burger, Ranch Fries, and Cole Slaw for lunch. Of course, Day 4 isn't bad either; you get Quesadillas and (the world's smallest piece of) Cheesecake. On Day 9 you get Breakfast Pizza in the morning and Cioppino for dinner, and on Day 5 there's Veal Marsala and Carrot Cake. On other days there's Lasagna, Poached Salmon, Lamb Chops Dijon, Lemon Frost, Tomato-Basil Ravioli, Barbecued Chicken, and . . .

As you can probably tell, we're proud of our menu at the Ranch. We think that our guests get a wide variety of delicious and interesting foods, well prepared and attractively served. We also think that they get something even more important: an education. Because we don't dictate what people eat, because we let them choose anything they want and as much as they want from the menu, we think they begin to understand the basics of what it means to eat well. Many follow our recommendations to the letter; others prefer to invent their own menu plans. Most of our guests lose weight while they're here, but weight loss is only one of the benefits we had in mind when we designed our menu.

It's true that there are no "bad" choices here, since we practice what we preach. All the dishes are low in fat, sugar, and salt and high in complex carbohydrates and fiber, and we limit protein to about six ounces a day. For guests who want to lose weight we suggest an intake of about 1000 calories a day for women and 1200 for men. We caution guests to eat more if they're extremely active, which most of them are. Still, just knowing the calorie counts of the food they ordered often opens people's eyes more than any lecture could. Of course, we don't have to serve cheesecake or any of the other sweet desserts; it would be easy and perfectly healthful to end each of the meals with fresh fruit. We serve those minuscule pieces of cake for a reason: we want people to see how big a piece of cake they should get used to eating is and learn to be satisfied with it. Not surprisingly, many guests would rather have a plate of fresh fruit.

What follows are recipes for some of the most popular dishes from our most recent 10-day menu cycle, including Pasta Marinara, Enid Zuckerman's favorite dish, and Vegetarian Chili, which is Mel's.

	DAY 1		DAY 2		DAY 3		DAY 4		DAY 5	
SHAKE	Blueberry	140	Carob	140	Strawberry	140	Orange	140	Banana	140
BREAKFAST	French Toast	110	Tropical Fruit		Bananas		Pasta Power	145	Danish	
	w/Pineapple-		w/Yogurt Sauce	85	Canyon Ranch	135			Rye Cereal	195
	Peach Butter	95	Bran Muffins	115	Canyon Ranch					
					Bread†	70				
LUNCH	Consomme	15	Antipasto Salad	115	Cold Blueberry		Fresh Carrot		Garlic Soup	40
	Curried Chicken				Soup	50	Soup	65		
	Salad in Pine-		Pizza†	260	Mandarin Salad	355	California		Bean Burrito†	280
	apple Boat		Truly Fruity	340	w/Roll	70	Tuna Salad	230	Fresh Fruit	40
	Banana Cake or	110	Cookie or	60	Custard	70	Fruit Kebab	55	or	
	Creole Vegetable†		Salade Nouvelle		or		or		Cold Poached	
	Gumbo	200	Fresh Fruit	40	Pita Pocket	240	Quesadilla	305	Salmon	225
	Fresh Fruit	40			Sandwich†	170	Cheesecake	95	Carob Cake	155
					Fresh Fruit	40				
DINNER	Pasta Salad	65	Carrot & Raisin		Salad of		Mixed Green		Fresh Tomato	
	Eggplant		Salad	60	Young Greens	60	Salad	15	Soup	75
	Florentine		Swordfish	235	w/Tarragon		Mexican		Veal Marsala*	240
	Baked Apple w/		Amandine*	140	Vinaigrette	20	Spaghetti†	290	Creamed Leeks	85
	Zabaglione		7-Grain Pilaf	65	Broiled Lobster		Fresh Vegetable	55	Wild Rice Pilaf	115
	Sauce*		Fresh Fruit	40	Tail†	40	Pear Crisp	60	Gingered Fruit	
	or		or		Scalloped		or		Compote w/	
	Fresh Fish†		Cheese		Potatoes	100	Lamb Chops		Cinnamon-Apple	
	Veracruz	130	Enchiladas†	130	Fresh Fruit	40	Dijon	270	Yogurt Sauce	90
	Rice Pilaf	110	Fantasy in Fruit	115	or		Fresh Fruit	40	or	
	Fresh Vegetable	30			Tamale Pie	200			Risotto w/	
	Fresh Fruit	40			Fresh Vegetable	55			Vegetables†	295
					Heavenly				Fresh Fruit	40
					Pudding	50				

Those desiring lower fat intake, choose
the entrees marked with a (†).

* Contains a trace of alcohol

10-DAY MENU (continued)

	DAY 6		DAY 7		DAY 8		DAY 9		DAY 10	
SHAKE	Blueberry	140	Orange	140	Strawberry	140	Peanut Butter	225	Banana	140
BREAKFAST	Fresh Fruit Blintz	 255	Melon Wedge Huevos Rancheros	45 135	7-Grain Waffle w/ Apple Butter & Fitness Cheese	 175	Breakfast Pizza Fresh Fruit	120 80	Oatmeal Pancake w/Fresh Fruit Jam	 155 25
LUNCH	Sherried Consomme* Canyon Ranch Stuft Spud Lemon Frost or Orzo Pasta† w/Seafood Fresh Fruit	 55 250 55 435 40	Miso Soup Cantonese Stir Fry† Rice Pudding or Warm Scallop Salad w/Raspberry Walnut Vinaigrette Fresh Fruit	50 350 135 245 40	Marinated Mushroom Salad White Chili w/Roll† Fresh Fruit or Artichoke Bowl w/Dilled Shrimp Whole Wheat Bagel Carrot Cake	 45 195 70 40 320 130	Canyon Ranch Guacamole Taco Salad w/Salsa Fresh Fruit or Egg Foo Yung w/Brown Rice, Pea Pods & Water Chestnuts† Blueberry Cheesecake	 60 310 30 40 105 95 75	Cole Slaw Canyon Ranch Burger w/sliced Tomato & Onion Ranch Fries Fresh Fruit or Ratatouille Au Gratin† Yogurt Parfait	60 190 110 40 220 110
DINNER	Minted Cucumber Salad Tomato-Basil Ravioli Pineapple Pie or Chicken Curry w/Chutney†* Fresh Fruit	 30 255 90 400 40	Lettuce & Fresh Herb Salad Steak au Poivre†* Baked Potato Skins Tomato Provencale Crepe Suzette* or Lasagna Fresh Fruit	 15 195 90 30 40 290 40	Spinach Salad w/Walnuts Paella Spanish Cream or Moroccan Chowder w/Couscous† Fresh Vegetable Fresh Fruit	 40 335 100 55 225 30 40	Italian Green Salad w/Croutons Cioppino* w/Garlic Bread† Fresh Fruit or Lentils Au Gratin Fresh Vegetable Fresh Fruit Sorbet	 40 335 200 95 40 225 30 25	Cold Pea Salad Barbecued Chicken Breast† Corn on the Cob Fresh Vegetable Fresh Fruit or Southwestern Vegetable Pie Pumpkin Tart	65 155 85 30 40 250 90

Those desiring lower fat intake, choose the entrees marked with a (†).

* Contains a trace of alcohol

INGREDIENTS

ORANGE SHAKE

EACH SERVING CONTAINS AP-PROXIMATELY:

138 CALORIES —16 CALORIES FROM FAT; 8 MG. CHOLESTEROL; 71 MG. SODIUM; .1 GM. FIBER

⅓ cup low-fat milk
2¼ teaspoons orange juice concentrate
¾ teaspoon vanilla extract
2¼ teaspoons nonfat dry milk
2¼ teaspoons fructose
½ cup ice

Combine all ingredients in a blender and blend until smooth.

Each recipe makes 1 (8-oz) serving

INGREDIENTS

BRAN MUFFINS

EACH MUFFIN CONTAINS AP-PROXIMATELY:

124 CALORIES —36 CALORIES FROM FAT; 21 MG. CHOLESTEROL; 197 MG. SODIUM; 4 GM. FIBER

1 cup whole wheat flour
1 teaspoon baking soda
¼ teaspoon salt
1½ cups unprocessed wheat bran
3 tablespoons melted corn oil margarine
¼ cup blackstrap molasses
1 egg, lightly beaten
1½ cups buttermilk
½ cup raisins

1 Preheat oven to 375 degrees. Spray muffin pans with nonstick vegetable coating.
2 Combine dry ingredients in a bowl and mix well.
3 In another bowl, combine other ingredients except raisins and mix well.
4 Add liquid ingredients to dry ingredients and stir just until dry ingredients are moistened. *Do not overmix.*
5 Stir in raisins and fill prepared muffin pans ¾ full.
6 Bake 15 to 20 minutes.

Makes 12 muffins

OATMEAL PANCAKES

EACH SERVING
CONTAINS
APPROXIMATELY:

155 CALORIES—1
CALORIE FROM FAT;
70 MG. CHOLESTEROL;
258 MG. SODIUM; 2
GM. FIBER

INGREDIENTS

2 cups rolled oat flour*
½ teaspoon salt
2 teaspoons baking powder
½ teaspoon baking soda
2 teaspoons fructose
2 teaspoons cinnamon
2 eggs
1 cup buttermilk
1 cup skim milk
2 tablespoons corn oil
1 cup Fresh Fruit Jam—(see page 255)

1 Sift all the dry ingredients together into a large bowl. In a medium mixing bowl combine all liquid ingredients and mix well.
2 Add liquid ingredients to dry ingredients and mix just until dry ingredients are moist (*Do not overmix*).
3 Use 2 tablespoons of batter for each pancake. Cook over medium heat until bubbles form on the surface and the under-side is lightly browned. Turn pancake over and cook on other side. Serve a stack of 4 pancakes with 2 tablespoons jam.

* Oat flour may be purchased in a health food store. If you can't find it, blend quick (*not instant*) dry oatmeal in blender to flour consistency.

Makes 8 (4 pancake) servings

INGREDIENTS

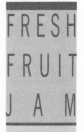

FRESH FRUIT JAM

1½ cups fresh fruit (you may use frozen as well)
1 tablespoon cornstarch
1 tablespoon water
2 teaspoons fructose

EACH SERVING
CONTAINS
APPROXIMATELY:

20 CALORIES—
1 CALORIE
FROM FAT; 0 MG.
CHOLESTEROL; 0
MG. SODIUM; 1
GM. FIBER

1   Heat fruit in saucepan over medium heat for approx-
    imately 3 minutes.
2   In a small bowl, mix cornstarch and water and stir
    into fruit.
3   Return to heat, add fructose, and whisk until thick.

Makes 12 (2 tablespoon) servings

INGREDIENTS

BREAKFAST PIZZA

4 whole-wheat English muffins, cut into halves
½ cup Fresh Fruit Jam—(see above)
1 cup grated part-skim mozzarella cheese (about 4 ounces)

EACH SERVING CON-
TAINS APPROXIMATELY:

152 CALORIES—49
CALORIES FROM FAT;
15 MG. CHOLESTEROL;
332 MG. SODIUM; 4 GM.
FIBER

1   Toast the muffin halves, cut sides up, under
    a broiler.
2   Spread 2 tablespoons jam on each muffin half;
    sprinkle ¼ cup grated cheese over the top of each.
3   Return to the broiler until the cheese is melted and
    very lightly browned. Serve immediately.

Makes 8 servings

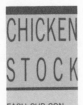

CHICKEN STOCK

EACH CUP CON-
TAINS APPROXI-
MATELY:

22 CALORIES—0
CALORIES FROM
FAT; 0 MG. CHO-
LESTEROL; 5 MG.
SODIUM; 0 GM.
FIBER

INGREDIENTS

2 to 4 pounds chicken bones, parts, and giblets
   (except the liver)
1 to 2 carrots, scraped and chopped
1 to 2 celery ribs without leaves, chopped
1 large onion cut into quarters
3 garlic cloves, cut into halves
1 bay leaf
12 whole peppercorns

1   Combine all ingredients in a large pot with a lid. Add cold water to cover and bring slowly to a boil.
2   Reduce heat, place cover slightly ajar to let steam escape, and simmer for 1 to 3 hours. The longer you cook the stock, the more flavorful it will be.
3   Cool to room temperature. Remove the chicken parts and vegetables and strain the stock. Refrigerate, uncovered, overnight or until the fat has hardened on the top.
4   Remove the fat and store the stock in the freezer in small containers.

Makes about 2 quarts

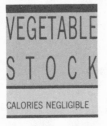

VEGETABLE STOCK

CALORIES NEGLIGIBLE

INGREDIENTS

1 small head cabbage, chopped
4 onions, chopped
6 carrots, scraped and chopped
1 small bunch celery without leaves, chopped
1 small bunch parsley, chopped
3 bay leaves
2 teaspoons dried marjoram, crushed
1 teaspoon salt
1 gallon water

1   Combine all ingredients in a large pot and bring to a boil. Reduce heat, cover, and simmer for 1 hour.
2   Strain the stock and refrigerate or store in the freezer in small containers.

<u>Makes about 3 quarts</u>

INGREDIENTS

EACH SERVING CONTAINS APPROXIMATELY:

30 CALORIES—2 CALORIES FROM FAT; 0 MG. CHOLESTEROL; 13 MG. SODIUM; .6 GM. FIBER

½ cup peeled and diced cucumbers
¾ cup diced red and green bell peppers
¾ cup diced onions
1 cup peeled and diced tomatoes
2½ cups tomato juice
2 minced garlic cloves or ½ teaspoon garlic powder
¼ teaspoon freshly ground black pepper
¼ teaspoon Worcestershire sauce
2 tablespoons freshly squeezed lemon juice
Chopped chives or green onion tops for garnish
2 lemons

1   In a large bowl, combine all ingredients except the chives or green onion tops and the lemon and mix thoroughly. Prepare a day in advance and chill.
2   Serve in chilled bowls and garnish with the chopped chives or green onion tops and a lemon wedge.

This recipe may also be used as a dip or as a sauce for a wide variety of salads, vegetables, and entrees.

<u>Makes 8 (½ cup) servings</u>

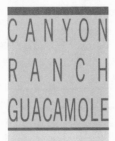

CANYON RANCH GUACAMOLE

EACH SERVING CONTAINS
APPROXIMATELY:

25 CALORIES—14 CALO-
RIES FROM FAT; 3 MG.
CHOLESTEROL; 154 MG.
SODIUM; 1 GM. FIBER

INGREDIENTS

2 cups chopped steamed asparagus
2¼ teaspoons lemon juice
3 tablespoons chopped onion
1 large tomato, chopped
¾ teaspoon salt (optional)
½ teaspoon chili powder
¼ teaspoon cumin
¼ teaspoon black pepper
¾ teaspoon minced garlic
  Dash tabasco sauce
⅓ cup sour cream
24 lettuce leaves
8 cherry tomatoes
36 tortilla chips

1   Add all ingredients except lettuce, tomatoes, and tortilla chips to blender container. Blend until smooth.
2   Transfer to bowl. Refrigerate several hours or overnight.
3   Line 12 salad plates with lettuce leaves. Add ¼ cup guacamole and garnish with one cherry tomato cut in half. Serve with 3 tortilla chips.

Makes 12 servings

CANYON RANCH DRESSING

EACH SERVING
CONTAINS APPROXI-
MATELY:

37 CALORIES—32
CALORIES FROM FAT;
0 MG. CHOLESTEROL;
123 MG. SODIUM; 0
GM. FIBER

INGREDIENTS

½ cup red wine vinegar
¼ teaspoon freshly ground black pepper
¾ teaspoon salt
2 teaspoons fructose
2 garlic cloves, minced
1½ teaspoons dried tarragon, crushed
1 teaspoon dried basil, crushed
¾ teaspoon dried oregano, crushed
2 teaspoons Worcestershire sauce
1 tablespoon Dijon mustard
  Juice of ½ lemon
¼ cup corn or safflower oil
1 cup water

Combine all ingredients except the water in a jar with a tight-fitting lid. Shake well. Add the water and shake well again. Refrigerate.
Note: The flavor is better if the dressing is made a day before you plan to use it.

Makes about 2 cups or 32 (2 tablespoon) servings

I N G R E D I E N T S

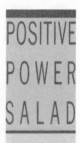

POSITIVE POWER SALAD

EACH SERVING CONTAINS APPROXIMATELY:

223 CALORIES—105 CALORIES FROM FAT; 10 MG. CHOLESTEROL; 134 MG. SODIUM; 4.1 GM. FIBER

⅓ cup raw sunflower seeds
2 cups chopped broccoli
2 cups sliced mushrooms
1½ cups chopped cauliflower
1½ cups diced jicama
1 cup diced carrots
½ cup diced yellow squash
½ cup diced zucchini
½ cup alfalfa sprouts
¼ cup finely chopped green onion tops
2 apples, diced
½ cup raisins
½ cup raw almonds, chopped
1 cup diced mozzarella cheese
¼ cup parmesan cheese, grated
¼ cup Canyon Ranch Dressing—(see page 258)

1 Toast the sunflower seeds and set aside.
2 Combine all other ingredients in a large bowl and mix thoroughly.
3 Divide into 8 servings. Sprinkle 2 teaspoons of toasted sunflower seeds over the top of each serving.

Makes 8 (1½ cup) servings

CURRIED CHICKEN SALAD IN PINEAPPLE BOAT

EACH SERVING CONTAINS APPROXIMATELY:

340 CALORIES—102 CALORIES FROM FAT; 72 MG. CHOLESTEROL; 235 MG. SODIUM; 2 GM. FIBER.

INGREDIENTS

2 fresh pineapples
6 cups cooked chicken breast, cut into bite-sized pieces
4 cups papaya, cut into bite-sized pieces
2 cups Curried Chutney Dressing—(see below)
Lettuce leaves
½ cup chopped, toasted walnuts

1 Quarter pineapples, leaving leaves attached. Remove pineapple from shell and cut into bite-sized pieces. Trim pineapple leaves with scissors. Set aside.
2 In a large bowl, combine chicken, papaya, pineapple, and dressing. Spoon 1⅔ cups of the mixture into each pineapple boat.
3 Line 8 chilled plates with lettuce leaves and place pineapple boat on each. Top with 1 tablespoon chopped walnuts.

Makes 8 servings

CURRIED CHUTNEY DRESSING

EACH SERVING CONTAINS APPROXIMATELY:

104 CALORIES—32 CALORIES FROM FAT; 1 MG. CHOLESTEROL; 113 MG. SODIUM, 1 GM. FIBER

INGREDIENTS

1½ cups reduced-calorie mayonnaise
1½ cups nonfat yogurt
2 tablespoons curry powder
¼ cup fructose
Pinch red pepper flakes
Pinch black pepper
1 teaspoon fresh minced garlic
¼ cup minced shallots
½ teaspoon Worcestershire sauce
1 teaspoon lemon juice
1 teaspoon low-sodium soy sauce
4 tablespoons red wine vinegar
1 cup Apple Chutney—(see page 261)

1 Combine all ingredients except Apple Chutney in a bowl. Stir until
   smooth.
2 Add Apple Chutney, mix well, cover, and refrigerate.

<u>Makes 16 (¼ cup) servings</u>

I N G R E D I E N T S

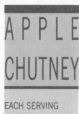

APPLE CHUTNEY

EACH SERVING
CONTAINS
APPROXIMATELY:

182 CALORIES—2
CALORIES FROM
FAT; 0 MG. CHOLES-
TEROL; 18 MG. SO-
DIUM; 1 GM. FIBER

  4 cups diced dried apples (dried without sulphur)
  1 cup finely diced dried figs
  1 cup finely diced golden raisins
  1 medium onion, finely chopped
1½ cups fructose or 2 cups sugar
1¼ teaspoons ground ginger
  ¼ cup pickling spice, tied in a cheesecloth bag
  2 cups water
  2 cups apple cider vinegar

1 Combine all ingredients in a large saucepan and bring to a boil. Reduce
   heat and simmer slowly, uncovered, for 2 hours.
2 Cool to room temperature. Remove and discard the cheesecloth bag.
   Refrigerate the chutney in a tightly covered container. It will keep for
   months.

<u>Makes 4¾ cups</u>

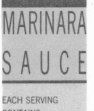

MARINARA SAUCE

EACH SERVING
CONTAINS
APPROXIMATELY:

75 CALORIES—18
CALORIES FROM FAT;
0 MG. CHOLESTEROL;
34 MG. SODIUM; 1
GM. FIBER

INGREDIENTS

1 cup onions
1 tablespoon minced garlic
½ cup Vegetable Stock (see page 256) or wine
1 teaspoon dried oregano, crushed
¾ teaspoon dried basil, crushed
1 bay leaf
½ teaspoon black pepper
2 cups sliced mushrooms
2¾ cups tomato sauce, no salt added
1¾ cups tomato purée, no salt added

1   In a large saucepan, sauté onions and garlic in stock or wine with crushed herbs, bay leaf, and black pepper until onions are tender. Add mushrooms and cook 5 minutes.
2   Add tomato products. Cover and simmer over low heat for 1 hour.

Makes 8 (½ cup) servings

THOUSAND ISLAND DRESSING

EACH SERVING CON-
TAINS APPROXIMATELY:

30 CALORIES—18 CAL-
ORIES FROM FAT; 0 MG.
CHOLESTEROL; 80 MG.
SODIUM; 1 GM. FIBER

INGREDIENTS

½ cup reduced-calorie mayonnaise
¼ cup bottled chili sauce
2 tablespoons sweet pickle relish
   Pinch salt
2 tablespoons red wine vinegar
   Pinch fructose
   Pinch black pepper
   Lemon juice to taste

1   Combine all ingredients in medium bowl and mix thoroughly.
2   Store covered in refrigerator.

Makes 8 (2 tablespoon) servings

I N G R E D I E N T S

2 small baking potatoes
1 medium onion, finely chopped
¼ cup buttermilk
½ cup lowfat cottage cheese
3 tablespoons grated parmesan or romano cheese
2 tablespoons chopped green onions, including the tops

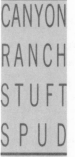

CANYON
RANCH
STUFT
SPUD

EACH SERVING
CONTAINS AP-
PROXIMATELY:

342 CALORIES
—32 CALORIES
FROM FAT; 12 MG.
CHOLESTEROL;
419 MG. SODIUM;
2 GM. FIBER

1   Wash the potatoes well. Pierce with the tines of a fork and bake at 400 degrees for 1 hour.
2   Cut a very thin slice from the top of each potato. Remove the pulp from the potatoes, being careful not to tear the shells. Mash the potato pulp and set aside in a covered bowl. Keep the shells warm.
3   Cook the onions, covered, over low heat until soft, stirring occasionally to prevent scorching. Add the mashed potatoes, cottage cheese, and all other ingredients except the chopped green onions. Mix well and heat thoroughly. Stuff the potato mixture back into the warm shells. They will be heaping way over the top.
4   To serve, sprinkle the top of each Stuft Spud with 1 tablespoon of chopped green onion. If you have prepared them in advance, heat in a 350 degree oven for 10 to 15 minutes before adding the chopped onions.

Makes 2 servings

INGREDIENTS

Sauce:
  1 onion, chopped
  2 cloves garlic, crushed
  ½ cup finely chopped parsley
  2 tablespoons Chicken Stock (see page 256)
  1 12-ounce can tomato paste
  1 teaspoon dried oregano, crushed
  ½ teaspoon dried basil, crushed
  ½ teaspoon salt
  ¼ teaspoon freshly ground black pepper
  2 Pizza Crusts (see page 265)
  2 large onions, thinly sliced
  1 pound mushrooms, thinly sliced
  1 small green bell pepper, sliced
  1 small red bell pepper, sliced
  2 small zucchini, thinly sliced
  1 pound sliced part-skim mozzarella cheese

PIZZA

EACH SERVING CONTAINS AP-PROXIMATELY:

274 CALORIES —80 CALORIES FROM FAT; 20 MG. CHOLES-TEROL; 405 MG. SODIUM; 5 GM. FIBER

1 Preheat oven to 425 degrees.
2 Sauté the onion, garlic, and parsley in the Chicken Stock until soft. Remove from heat and add tomato paste, oregano, basil, salt, and black pepper. Mix thoroughly.
3 Spread half of the sauce over each of the two pizza crusts. Arrange onions, mushrooms, pepper slices, and zucchini on top. Bake 10 minutes on the lowest shelf of the oven.
4 Place cheese slices on pizzas and bake for an additional 15 minutes. Allow pizza to stand for 3 to 5 minutes before slicing. If pizza begins to brown too much before the crust is done, place a square of aluminum foil lightly over top. Continue baking until the bottom crust is lightly browned. Cut each pizza into 6 slices.

Makes 12 servings

INGREDIENTS

1 package active dry yeast
1 cup warm water
3 cups whole wheat flour
1 tablespoon olive oil
½ teaspoon salt

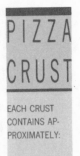

PIZZA
CRUST

EACH CRUST
CONTAINS AP-
PROXIMATELY:

670 CALORIES—
95 CALORIES
FROM FAT; 0 MG.
CHOLESTEROL;
560 MG. SODIUM;
22 GM. FIBER

1   Soften yeast in warm water. Add 1½ cups of flour and mix well. Add olive oil and salt and stir until mixed.

2   Add another cup of flour and mix. Place on floured board and knead until smooth and elastic (10 to 15 minutes), adding the remaining ½ cup flour if needed.

3   Place in an oiled bowl and turn dough so that the oiled side is up. Cover dough with waxed paper or plastic wrap. Put in a warm place for 1½ to 2 hours, until it is doubled in bulk. Punch down. Refrigerate until cold.

4   Divide dough in half and roll out on a lightly floured board. Place in two 12-inch pizza pans. (If you are not going to make pizza immediately, wrap and freeze. Thaw completely before placing sauce, toppings, and cheese over the top.)

5   To finish pizza see Pizza recipe.

Makes two 12-inch pizza crusts

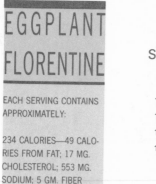

EGGPLANT FLORENTINE

EACH SERVING CONTAINS
APPROXIMATELY:

234 CALORIES—49 CALO-
RIES FROM FAT; 17 MG.
CHOLESTEROL; 553 MG.
SODIUM; 5 GM. FIBER

INGREDIENTS

Sauce:
 1 quart skim milk
 3 tablespoons corn oil margarine
 ⅓ cup flour
 ¼ teaspoon salt
 ¼ teaspoon white pepper
 ¼ teaspoon nutmeg
 1 cup part-skim Swiss cheese

1 To make sauce, heat milk in top of double boiler. Melt margarine in another pan and add flour. Cook 3 minutes.
2 Add flour mixture to simmering milk and cook, stirring until thickened (about 15 minutes).
3 Add salt, white pepper, nutmeg, and Swiss cheese and stir until cheese is melted completely. Set sauce aside.

Eggplant and spinach:
 2 medium eggplants, peeled
12 cups fresh spinach, chopped
 4 cups sauce
 ½ cup freshly grated parmesan cheese

1 Blanch spinach by steaming for 1 minute.
2 Slice eggplants crosswise into ¼-inch-thick rounds. Place in glass baking dish and sprinkle liberally with salt. Cover and let stand 1 hour. Rinse salt off each round and pat dry with a paper towel. Rinse dish. Steam eggplant until it can be easily pierced with a fork, about 4 minutes.
3 Line the bottom of 8 au gratin dishes with half the spinach. Divide eggplant and place equal amounts over each dish of spinach, then place the rest of spinach on top of eggplant. Pour ½ cup sauce over each and sprinkle with 1 tablespoon parmesan cheese. Bake for 20 to 30 minutes at 350 degrees.

Makes 8 servings

I N G R E D I E N T S

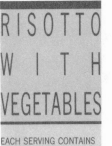

RISOTTO WITH VEGETABLES

EACH SERVING CONTAINS
APPROXIMATELY:

290 CALORIES—46 CALO-
RIES FROM FAT; 6 MG.
CHOLESTEROL; 350 MG.
SODIUM; 3 GM. FIBER

1½ tablespoons olive oil
  2 cups finely chopped onions
 ⅓ cup finely chopped parsley
  1 cup finely chopped celery
  2 tablespoons finely chopped fresh basil
  2 teaspoons finely chopped garlic
  2 cups long-grain brown rice
  1 cup lentils
  5 cups Vegetable Stock (see page 256) or water
  1 pound mushrooms, sliced
  2 carrots, julienned
  1 each, red and green bell peppers, julienned
 12 asparagus stalks
  1 cup skim milk
  2 tablespoons cream of rice
  1 teaspoon salt
 ¼ teaspoon black pepper
  1 cup parmesan cheese

1 In a large covered pot, heat oil and add onions, parsley, celery, basil, and
   garlic. Sauté until onions are golden. Add rice, lentils, and stock or
   water. Cover and bring to a boil. Reduce heat and simmer about 40
   minutes or until rice and lentils are tender.
2 Keeping mushrooms separate, steam vegetables until crisp-tender. Set
   aside.
3 In a small pan bring milk to a boil and add cream of rice, salt, and
   pepper. Stir for 30 seconds, remove from heat and cover. Set aside for 5
   minutes. Transfer mixture to a blender and purée. Add cheese and
   continue to blend.
4 When rice is done, add cheese mixture, all of the mushrooms, and 2 cups
   vegetable mixture. Mix thoroughly.
5 To serve, spoon 1 cup rice mixture into dish and top with ½ cup julienned
   vegetables.

Makes 8 (1½ cup) servings

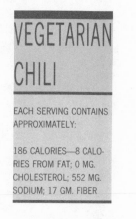

VEGETARIAN CHILI

EACH SERVING CONTAINS
APPROXIMATELY:

186 CALORIES—8 CALO-
RIES FROM FAT; 0 MG.
CHOLESTEROL; 552 MG.
SODIUM; 17 GM. FIBER

I N G R E D I E N T S

1½ cups finely chopped onions
 ½ tablespoon minced fresh garlic
 ⅓ cup chopped canned green chilies, undrained
 1 cup diced tomatoes
 ½ teaspoon Vegit
 1 teaspoon oregano
 1 teaspoon cumin
1¼ teaspoons chili powder
 3 cups canned red kidney beans, drained
1½ cups tomato juice, no salt added
   Cheddar cheese (optional)

1   Combine the onion and garlic in a large skillet or saucepan and cook, covered, over low heat until soft, stirring frequently to prevent scorching.
2   Add all other ingredients and mix thoroughly.
3   Cook over medium heat until bubbling and hot.
4   If you like, sprinkle 2 tablespoons grated cheddar cheese over the top of each serving.

Makes 5 (1 cup) servings

MEXICAN SPAGHETTI

EACH SERVING CON-
TAINS APPROXIMATELY:

55 CALORIES—2 CALO-
RIES FROM FAT; 0 MG.
CHOLESTEROL; 313
MG. SODIUM; 1 GM.
FIBER

I N G R E D I E N T S

1 cup finely chopped onion
2 minced garlic cloves
1 28-ounce can low-sodium solid pack tomatoes
1 6-ounce can low-sodium tomato paste
¾ cup water
¼ cup red wine
1 teaspoon fructose
1 stalk celery, finely chopped
2 tablespoons chopped cilantro
1 teaspoon salt
¼ teaspoon freshly ground black pepper
1 bay leaf
¾ teaspoon cumin
1½ teaspoons chili powder
½ teaspoon dried thyme, crushed
½ teaspoon dried oregano, crushed
2 dashes Tabasco

11 Combine the onion and garlic in a heavy pan and cook, covered, over very low heat until the vegetables are transparent. Add stock or water, if necessary, to prevent scorching.

2 In another pan, combine tomatoes, tomato paste, water, and wine. Bring to a boil and then reduce heat to simmer. Add onion mixture, fructose, celery, and all seasonings.

3 Cover and simmer for 1 hour, adding stock or water if too thick.

4 Serve over your choice of pasta.

Makes 8 (½ cup) servings

INGREDIENTS

1 cup chopped onion
1 cup chopped green bell pepper, seeded
¼ cup chopped green onion tops
1 teaspoon minced garlic
2 tablespoons Chicken Stock (see page 256)
½ cup chopped parsley
3 cups tomato sauce (no salt added)
1 cup water
1 cup dry white wine
1 teaspoon salt
½ teaspoon ground black pepper
¼ teaspoon dried rosemary
¼ teaspoon dried thyme
1 bay leaf
¾ pound firm white fish, cubed
¾ pound large shrimp or prawns
8 clams in the shell

CIOPPINO

EACH SERVING CONTAINS APPROXIMATELY:

199 CALORIES—21 CALORIES FROM FAT; 56 MG. CHOLESTEROL; 414 MG. SODIUM; 1 GM. FIBER

1 In a large saucepan, sauté the onions, bell pepper, green onions, and garlic in stock until tender.

2 Add parsley, tomato sauce, water, wine, and pepper. Crush rosemary and thyme with a mortar and pestle and add with bay leaf. Cover and simmer for one hour.

3 Add the cubed fish and shrimp and cook for 5 to 10 minutes.

4 Steam clams separately until they open, 5 to 10 minutes.

5 Serve in large bowls with a clam on top of each serving.

Makes 8 (1½ cup) servings

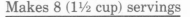

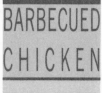

BARBECUED CHICKEN

EACH SERVING CONTAINS
APPROXIMATELY:

132 CALORIES—30 CALO-
RIES FROM FAT; 53 MG.
CHOLESTEROL; 192 MG.
SODIUM; .3 GM. FIBER

INGREDIENTS

8 chicken legs
  Garlic powder
Sauce:
  1 large onion, minced
  1 8-ounce can low-sodium tomato sauce
  ¼ cup freshly squeezed lemon juice
  3 tablespoons Worcestershire sauce
  2 tablespoons white vinegar
  2 tablespoons fructose
1½ teaspoons dry mustard
  ¼ teaspoon salt
  1 cup water
  ½ teaspoon Liquid Smoke

1   Preheat oven to 350 degrees. Place the chicken legs in a baking dish and sprinkle lightly with garlic powder. Cover the baking dish with a lid or aluminum foil and bake for 30 minutes.

2   Remove chicken legs from the oven and cool until they can be handled easily.

3   To make sauce, sauté the onions in a nonstick pan until they are soft.

4   Combine the tomato sauce, lemon juice, Worcestershire sauce, and vinegar in a bowl. Add the fructose, dry mustard, and salt and mix thoroughly. Add mixture and 1 cup of water to the onions. Mix well and slowly bring to a boil. Cover and simmer for ½ hour.

5   Remove from the heat and add the Liquid Smoke. Mix well. Use immediately or cool to room temperature and store, covered, in the refrigerator.

6   When chicken is cool, remove and discard the skin and place the chicken legs back in the dish.

7   Pour ¼ cup of the sauce over each chicken leg. Cover and bake for 20 minutes more.

Makes 8 servings

INGREDIENTS

8 small loin lamb chops (all fat removed), cut 1½ inch thick
Garlic powder
Freshly ground black pepper
3 cups parsley, finely chopped
3 tablespoons unprocessed wheat bran
¾ cup Dijon mustard

1 Preheat oven to 500 degrees.
2 Lightly sprinkle both sides of the lamb chops with
   garlic powder and freshly ground black pepper and
   place them in a baking dish.
3 Combine the parsley, wheat bran, and mustard and
   mix thoroughly.
4 Spread the mustard mixture evenly over the tops
   of the lamb chops.
5 Place in the center of oven for 4 minutes. Turn the
   oven off but do not open the door for 30 more minutes.

Makes 8 servings

LAMB CHOPS DIJON

EACH SERVING CONTAINS APPROXIMATELY:

144 CALORIES —53 CALORIES FROM FAT; 57 MG. CHOLESTEROL; 716 MG. SODIUM; .8 GM. FIBER

INGREDIENTS

1 pound lean ground beef
8 small whole-wheat buns
⅓ cup Thousand Island Dressing
Tomato and onion slices
Lettuce

1 Form the beef into eight 2-ounce patties and cook
   as desired.
2 Spread each bun with 2 teaspoons dressing.
3 Place the patty on the bun. Garnish with tomato,
   onion slices, and lettuce.

Makes 8 burgers

CANYON RANCH BURGER

EACH SERVING CONTAINS APPROXIMATELY:

221 CALORIES —77 CALORIES FROM FAT; 54 MG. CHOLESTEROL; 101 MG. SODIUM; 2 GM. FIBER

**RANCH
FRIES**

EACH SERVING
CONTAINS AP-
PROXIMATELY:

62 CALORIES
—0 CALORIES
FROM FAT; 0
MG. CHOLES-
TEROL; 5 MG.
SODIUM; 1 GM.
FIBER

INGREDIENTS

4 baking potatoes, cut into strips

1 Preheat oven to 375 degrees.
2 Spread fries on a large baking sheet sprayed heavily
   with nonstick vegetable coating. Do not overlap.
   Spray tops of potato strips lightly with nonstick
   vegetable coating.
3 Bake for 1 hour, turning over at 15-minute intervals.

Makes 12 servings

INGREDIENTS

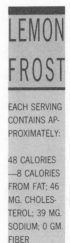

LEMON FROST

EACH SERVING CONTAINS APPROXIMATELY:

48 CALORIES
—8 CALORIES FROM FAT; 46 MG. CHOLESTEROL; 39 MG. SODIUM; 0 GM. FIBER

2 egg whites (room temperature)
½ cup water
½ cup nonfat dry milk
2 egg yolks
¼ cup fructose
¼ teaspoon lemon peel
⅛ teaspoon salt
¼ cup lemon juice
　Mint sprigs and lemon wheels

1　With electric mixer, beat egg whites, water, and dry milk in a small bowl until soft peaks form. Scrape bowl frequently to make sure the dry milk dissolves.

2　In a separate bowl, beat remaining ingredients together until fructose is completely dissolved. Gradually beat mix into the whipped egg whites.

3　Spoon into individual dessert dishes and freeze for at least 2 hours or until solid.

4　Garnish with mint sprigs and lemon wheels.

<u>Makes 6 servings</u>

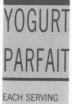

YOGURT PARFAIT

EACH SERVING CONTAINS AP- PROXIMATELY:

110 CALORIES —14 CALORIES FROM FAT; 2 MG. CHOLESTEROL; 88 MG. SODIUM; 0 GM. FIBER

I N G R E D I E N T S

1 tablespoon corn oil margarine
1 tablespoon all-purpose flour
1 cup water
4 tablespoons carob powder
1 teaspoon dry decaffeinated coffee
2 tablespoons fructose
2 tablespoons vanilla extract
1 quart plain nonfat yogurt

1 Melt margarine in saucepan. Add flour and stir over medium heat for approximately 2 minutes.
2 Bring water to a boil. Add carob, fructose, and coffee, stirring continuously. Add this to flour mixture. Heat and stir until it thickens.
3 Remove pan from heat and add vanilla. Cool slightly.
4 Scoop ½ cup yogurt into a sherbet glass and top with 2 tablespoons of sauce.

Makes 8 servings

I N G R E D I E N T S

1 cup raisins
½ cup chopped dried apricots
½ cup chopped pitted dates
½ cup chopped walnuts
1 cup whole wheat flour
¼ cup corn oil
1 tablespoon vanilla extract
¼ teaspoon salt
2 eggs
1 16-ounce can unsweetened, crushed pineapple, drained

TRULY FRUITY COOKIE

EACH SERVING CONTAINS AP-PROXIMATELY:

70 CALORIES— 26 CALORIES FROM FAT; 15 MG. CHOLES-TEROL; 22 MG. SODIUM; 1 GM. FIBER

1 Preheat oven to 350 degrees. Spray a 9- × 5-inch bread pan with nonstick vegetable coating.
2 Combine raisins, apricots, dates, walnuts, and flour in a large bowl and mix well. Set aside.
3 In another bowl, combine all other ingredients and mix well. Add liquid ingredients to fruit mixture and stir thoroughly.
4 Pour into prepared bread pan and bake for 1 hour or until a toothpick inserted in center comes out clean. Remove from oven to a rack and cool to room temperature. Cut into 1-inch slices and then into quarters.

Makes 36 servings

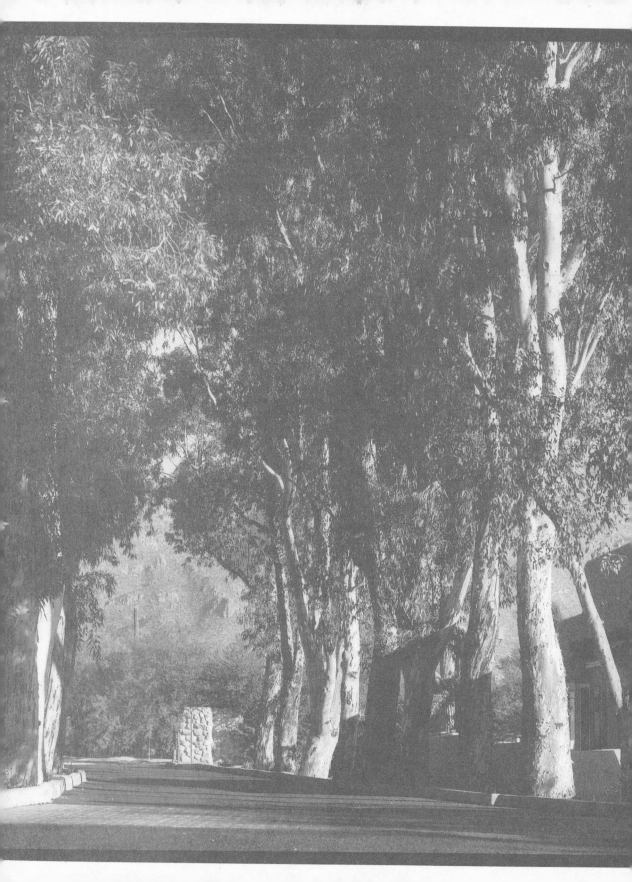

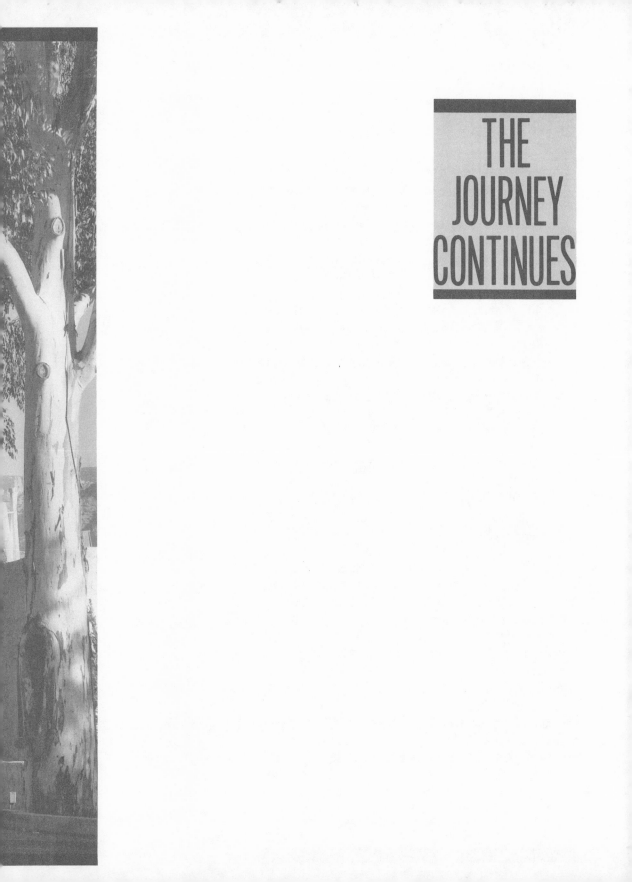

THE JOURNEY CONTINUES

AFTERWORD

■

J ust as we were putting the finishing touches
on this book, I reached another landmark
birthday, my sixtieth. It was a sentimental
occasion, and I couldn't help but spend time
during the days leading up to the event
reflecting long and hard about my life, my work
here at the Ranch, and my continuing journey to
wellness.

On the Big Day my wife Enid threw me a "This
Is Your Life" surprise party. The room was filled
with family and old and dear friends, and the
walls were lined with huge blown-up photographs
of me throughout my life: as a baby, as a grammar
school student, as a skinny teenager, as a navy
reservist, all the way up to today. In the middle of
the party one of my old high-school buddies asked
me a question that gave me pause. "Doesn't it
depress you to see yourself looking so young in all
these pictures?" he asked.

I have to admit that once in a while I feel a tiny
tug of nostalgia for my old hairline and my
unlined face, but my answer to my old friend was
an unqualified and resounding *no*. I feel better—
healthier, happier, and more fulfilled—today than
I did when any of those pictures was taken. I
haven't stopped the clock, but I have slowed it
down. I'll never know for sure if my lifestyle
changes over the last decade have added years to
my life (although I certainly believe they have);
I'm positive, however, that my new habits have
added life to my years.

As I read this book one final time, I was reminded of a story that my colleague Bill Day tells
about a 45-year-old woman he worked with when
he was fitness director of a spa in Houston several
years ago. Bill helped the woman create an exercise program, and during the two weeks she spent
at the spa he monitored her progress and got to

know her quite well. She absolutely flourished during her visit; she relaxed for the first time in years, lost six pounds, lowered her blood pressure, and fell in love with racewalking.

On the morning of the day the woman was scheduled to return home, Bill caught up with her on the jogging track and asked how she was feeling. "Well, actually I'm a little depressed," she responded. "I'm going to Paris on vacation next month, and I just know I'm going to eat and drink too much and not get enough exercise while I'm there."

Bill thought for a moment and said, "But how do you feel now, right this minute?"

Her answer was immediate and brimming over with passion: "I feel better today than I have ever felt in my life!"

"Well," said Bill, "isn't it great to know that you're never more than two weeks away from feeling better than you've ever felt in your life?"

I think about that story often, especially now that I have the Canyon Ranch program summed up in a large stack of manuscript paper in front of me. What we tell our guests at Canyon Ranch is all here in these pages. The only ingredient missing is the most important one of all: your commitment.

There are only so many hours in the day, and for most people those days are chockful already. If you add something, anything, to your daily schedule, you are probably going to have to subtract something else. You have to decide what's important in your life and act on that decision. No matter what you decide to do, vow to accept yourself for what you are, imperfect perhaps but ultimately in charge of your own life. If you can't make all the changes you'd like, don't put your life on hold, saying that as soon as you lose weight or quit smoking or start going to aerobics class, your life will be back on track again. Self-acceptance is a vital component of health and happiness.

The truth is, you don't change your life by reading a book or even by visiting a spa. You do it by caring enough about yourself to take responsibility for your health and well-being. Only you can make the decision to fuel and move your body so that it stays healthy. Only you can give yourself time to reflect, relax, and dream.

I and Enid and everyone else here at Canyon Ranch hope you will choose to find out how good it feels to be healthy. I guarantee you it will change your life.

—M. Z.

INDEX

(Page numbers in *italics* refer to recipes.)

ABOUT THE AUTHORS

The Canyon Ranch Staff is composed of doctors, nurses, exercise physiologists, registered dietitians, psychologists, wellness counselors, skin care specialists, and massage therapists—all fit, all knowledgeable, and all brimming with enthusiasm. These experts have provided the information in **The Canyon Ranch Health and Fitness Program.**

Kathleen Moloney has written, or co-written, several books, including *40 Plus for Women, Baseball by the Rules, Ventriloquism for the Total Dummy,* and *Esquire Etiquette.* She lives in New York City.

Canyon Ranch
8600 E. Rockcliff Road
Tucson, Arizona 85715
1-800-742-9000   USA
1-800-327-9090   Canada
1-602-749-9000   Worldwide